T0301215

Basic Theories of Traditional Chinese Medicine

Companion volumes

Diagnostics of Traditional Chinese Medicine
Edited by Zhu Bing and Wang Hongcai
ISBN 978 1 84819 036 8
International Acupuncture Textbooks

Meridians and Acupoints
Edited by Zhu Bing and Wang Hongcai
ISBN 978 1 84819 037 5
International Acupuncture Textbooks

Acupuncture Therapeutics
Edited by Zhu Bing and Wang Hongcai
ISBN 978 1 84819 039 9
International Acupuncture Textbooks

Case Studies from the Medical Records of Leading Chinese Acupuncture Experts
Edited by Zhu Bing and Wang Hongcai
ISBN 978 1 84819 046 7
International Acupuncture Textbooks

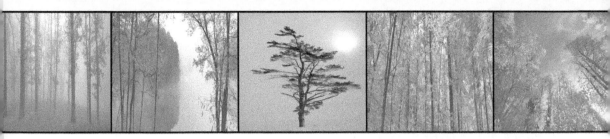

International
Acupuncture
Textbooks

Basic Theories of Traditional Chinese Medicine

Chief Editors: Zhu Bing and Wang Hongcai

Advisor: Cheng Xinnong

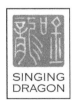

SINGING
DRAGON

London and Philadelphia

China Beijing International Acupuncture Training Center
Institute of Acupuncture and Moxibustion
China Academy of Chinese Medical Sciences
Advisor: Cheng Xinnong
Chief Editors: Zhu Bing, Wang Hongcai
Deputy Editors: Hu Xuehua, Huang Hui, Yu Min, Wang Huizhu
Members of the Editorial Board: Huang Hui, Hong Tao, Hu Xuehua, Liu Xuan, Liu Yuting,
Wang Fang, Wang Hongcai, Wang Huizhu, Wang Yue, Wu Mozheng, Yu Min, Zhu Bing,
Zhang Nan, Zhang Yi

First published in 2010
by Singing Dragon (an imprint of Jessica Kingsley Publishers)
in co-operation with People's Military Medical Press
116 Pentonville Road
London N1 9JB, UK
and
400 Market Street, Suite 400
Philadelphia, PA 19106, USA

Library of Congress Cataloging in Publication Data
A CIP catalog record for this book is available from the Library of Congress

British Library Cataloguing in Publication Data
A CIP catalogue record for this book is available from the British Library

ISBN 978 1 84819 038 2

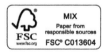

CHINA BEIJING INTERNATIONAL ACUPUNCTURE TRAINING CENTER

China Beijing International Acupuncture Training Center (CBIATC) was set up in 1975 at the request of the World Health Organization (WHO) and with the approval of the State Council of the People's Republic of China. Since its foundation, it has been supported and administered by WHO, the Chinese government, the State Administration of Traditional Chinese Medicine (SATCM) and the China Academy of Chinese Medical Sciences (CACMS). Now it has developed into a world-famous, authoritative training organization.

Since 1975, aiming to popularize acupuncture to the world, CBIATC has been working actively to accomplish the task, 'to perfect ways of acupuncture training and provide more opportunities for foreign doctors', assigned by WHO. More than 30 years' experience has created an excellent teaching team led by the academician, Professor Cheng Xinnong, and a group of professors. The multiple courses here are offered in different languages, including English, German, Spanish and Japanese. According to statistics, so far CBIATC has provided training in acupuncture, Tuina Massage, Traditional Chinese Medicine, Qigong, and so on for over 10,000 medical doctors and students from 106 countries and regions.

The teaching programmes of CBIATC include three-month and various short courses, are carefully and rationally worked out based on the individual needs of participants. Characterized by the organic combination of theory with practice, there are more than ten cooperating hospitals for the students to practice in. With professional teaching and advanced services, CBIATC will lead you to the profound and wonderful world of acupuncture.

Official website: www.cbiatc.com
Training support: www.tcmoo.com

PREFACE

More than 2000 years ago, a Chinese doctor named Bianque saved the life of a crown prince simply with an acupuncture needle. The story became one of the earliest acupuncture medical cases and went down in history. It is perhaps since then that people have been fascinated by the mystery of acupuncture and kept on studying it. In 1975, at the request of the World Health Organization, an acupuncture school was founded in Beijing, China, namely the China Beijing International Acupuncture Training Center. As one of the sponsor institutions, the Center compiled a textbook of Chinese Acupuncture and Moxibustion for foreign learners, published in 1980 and reprinted repeatedly afterwards, which has been of profound, far-reaching influence. It has been adopted as a 'model book' for acupuncture education and examination in many countries, and has played a significant role in the global dissemination of acupuncture.

Today, with the purpose of extending this 'authentic and professional' knowledge, we have compiled a series of books entitled *International Acupuncture Textbooks* to introduce incisively the basic theories of Traditional Chinese Medicine (TCM) and acupuncture–moxibustion techniques, by building on and developing the characteristics of the original textbook of Chinese Acupuncture and Moxibustion; and presenting authoritatively the systematic teaching materials with concise explanation based on a core syllabus for TCM professional education in China.

In addition, just as the same plant might have its unique properties when growing in different geographical environments, this set of books may reflect, in its particular style, our experience accumulated over 30 years of international acupuncture training.

Zhu Bing and Wang Hongcai

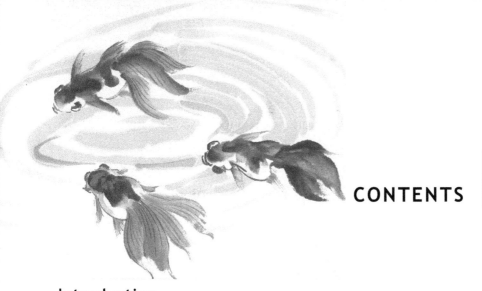

CONTENTS

CHAPTER 5 The Aetiology and Occurrence of Diseases.... 117

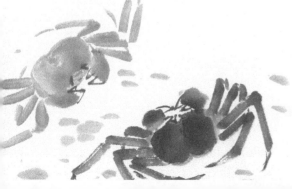

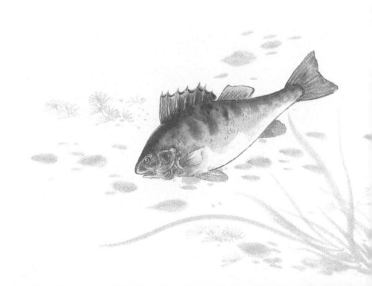

INTRODUCTION

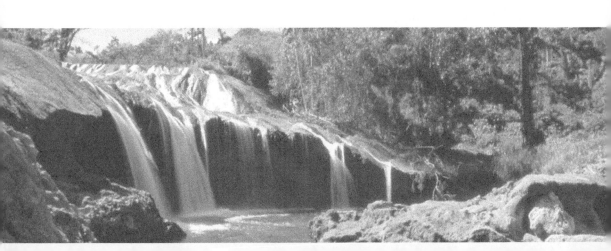

I. THE ORIGIN AND DEVELOPMENT OF TRADITIONAL CHINESE MEDICINE (TCM)

1. FORMATION OF THE THEORETICAL SYSTEMS OF TCM

The period of formation: The origins of the formulation of TCM date from the Spring and Autumn period and Warring States period through to the Qin and Han dynasties.

Huangdi's Internal Classic, the earliest extant medical classic in China, established the unique theoretical systems of TCM and laid a foundation for its development.

Significance: *Huangdi's Internal Classic* is made up of two parts: *Plain Questions* (available in several English translations) and *Miraculous Pivot*. There are 81 chapters in each part.

Based on the Theory of Yin–Yang and Five Elements and its holistic concept, it explains the general laws of the functional activities of the body, the relationship of the human body to nature and the natural environment. It explains in systematic terms the anatomical structures of the body, the Zang Fu organs, meridians and collaterals, physiology and pathology, and other aspects of diagnosis, prevention and treatment of diseases. It further addresses important philosophical concepts such as the nature of Qi, and the relationship between heaven and man, body and Mind.

2. WRITTEN DEVELOPMENT OF THE THEORETICAL SYSTEMS OF TCM

2.1 Before the Han dynasty

Classic on Medical Problems, written by Qin Yueren, supplemented *Huangdi's Internal Classic* and laid a further foundation for TCM theories.

2.2 The Han dynasty

Treatise on Febrile and Miscellaneous Diseases, written by Zhang Zhongjing at the end of the Eastern Han dynasty, was the first clinical medical book, in which the method of treatment based on syndrome differentiation was emphasized. Later, in the Jin dynasty, the book was revised into two books: *Treatise on Febrile Diseases* and *Synopsis of Prescriptions from the Golden Chamber* by Wang Shuhe, a medical doctor.

2.3 The Jin and Sui dynasties

Treatment of Different Kinds of Diseases, written by Chao Yuanfang in the Sui dynasty, was the first medical work about aetiology, pathogenesis and syndrome analysis.

2.4 The Song, Jin, Yuan dynasties

Key to Therapeutics of Children's Diseases, the earliest paediatric monograph extant in China, was written by Qian Yi in the Song dynasty.

Prescriptions Assigned to the Three Categories of Pathogenic Factors of Diseases, written by Chen Wuze in the Song dynasty, put forward the theory of 'three causes' as far as the aetiology was concerned.

Well-known physicians of the four schools of the Jin-Yuan dynasty:

- **Liu Wansu** (the school of cooling) emphasized the usage of 'herbal drugs cold and cool in nature' because the 'six exogenous factors all arise from Fire' and 'five emotions in excess would turn into Fire'.

- **Zhang Congzheng** (the school of purgation) believed that all diseases were caused by 'evil factors'. Once the pathogenic factors were expelled, the normal conditions of the body would naturally be restored. His methods of removing evils included diaphoresis, emesis and purgation.

- **Li Gao** (the school of strengthening the Spleen and Stomach) thought that diseases, apart from external causes, were mainly brought about by internal injury of the Spleen and Stomach, and advocated cure by building up and regulating the Spleen and Stomach.

- **Zhu Danxi** (the school of nourishing Yin) said 'the body often has more than enough Yang but not enough Yin'. So, he emphasized the principle of nourishing Yin and reducing Fire for treatment of diseases.

2.5 The Ming and Qing dynasties

Treatise on Pestilence was written by Wu Youke in the Ming dynasty. He was the first person who put forward the theory of 'pestilential Qi' and believed that the infectious epidemic diseases were caused neither by Wind, Cold, Summer Heat nor Damp, but a kind of evil Qi in nature that invaded the body through the mouth and nose rather than from the body surface. His idea brought about a breakthrough in the development of aetiology for infectious febrile diseases.

Ye Tianshi and Wu Jutong were famous physicians of the Qing dynasty who developed the method of diagnosis and treatment for epidemic febrile diseases by establishing the differentiation of syndromes according to the Theory of Wei (defence), Qi (vital energy), Ying (nutrient) and Xue (Blood), and the Theory of Sanjiao (Triple Burner), so as to systematize the theoretical systems of aetiology, pathogenesis, pulse diagnosis, syndrome differentiation and treatment for febrile diseases.

Corrections on the Errors of Medical Works was written by Wang Qingren in the Qing dynasty. His emphasis was on the anatomy and he corrected anatomical errors in the medical classics. Furthermore, he developed the theory that Blood stasis could cause diseases, and also presented methods of treatment for syndromes caused by Blood stagnation.

II. THE BASIC CHARACTERISTICS OF TCM

1. THE HOLISTIC CONCEPT

TCM views the human body as an organic whole, and the relationship between the human being and nature as an integral unity. As an organic whole, the various parts of the body are inseparable in structure; the organs are related physiologically and influenced pathologically. This holistic concept includes two aspects: the human body as an organic whole, and the unity between the human body and nature.

1.1 The human body as an organic whole

Taking the five Zang organs as a core, all parts of the body including the six Fu organs, five tissues, five sense organs, four limbs, are related to each other, linked via meridians and collaterals. They complete the body's functional activities through the actions of Essence, Qi, Blood and Body Fluid.

1.2 The unity between the human body and nature

Seasonal and climatic influence on the body: In spring and summer, it is warm and hot, so Yang Qi disperses. The skin of the body is relaxed, the pores are open and there is sweating. The body clears Heat through sweating to regulate the balance of Yin and Yang. In autumn and winter, it is Cold, Yang Qi is stored, the skin of the body remains tight, the pores closed, there is less sweat, but more urine to ensure normal water metabolism, signifying the body's adaptability to the physiological adjustment.

Day and night influence on the human body: Yang Qi of the body circulates externally during the day and remains in the exterior to promote the functional activities of the Zang Fu organs. In the morning, Yang Qi starts to rise; at noon, Yang Qi becomes flourishing, and at night, Yang Qi tends to be kept inside to let people sleep. This reflects the process of the decrease and increase of Yin and Yang during the day and at night, and the changes to the physiological functional activities.

Geographical influence on the human body: TCM holds that geographical difference, including climatic difference in different regions, living environment, and custom, will affect the physiological activities of the body to a certain degree. When one moves to a new place, one might not be used to the climate and environment at first. However, the body is able to make the relevant adjustment and one gets used to the change after a time.

2. TREATMENT BASED ON DIFFERENTIATION OF SYNDROMES

This is a basic principle, as well as a special method and one of the defining characteristics of TCM, used to analyze and treat diseases.

2.1 Syndrome

A syndrome can be described as an overall summary of the pathological changes at a certain stage in the course of a disease, which takes in the location, cause, nature of the disease, describes the relationship between the antipathogenic Qi and pathogenic factors, and reflects the pathological changes in a certain period of time in the course of the development of the diseases. So the term 'syndrome' implies a more comprehensive assessment of a disease than a mere description of symptoms.

2.2 Differentiation of syndromes

Differentiation of syndromes defines the procedure for identifying a patient's condition. Through the synthesis of relevant information provided by the four diagnostic methods, the cause, nature, location and relationship between the antipathogenic Qi and pathogenic factors, the root cause of the disease can be identified.

Treatment based on differentiation of syndromes

The method and principle of treatment are worked out according to the result of syndrome differentiation.

Relationship between syndrome differentiation and treatment based on differentiation of syndromes

Syndrome differentiation is a necessary prerequisite for deciding on appropriate treatment, while treatment based on differentiation of syndromes is a method used to treat a disease. In fact, the success of syndrome differentiation can be proven by the therapeutic effect of the treatment. The procedure of differentiating syndromes and giving treatment based on syndrome differentiation is the process of analyzing and treating the diseases.

2.3 Relationship between differentiation of diseases and differentiation of syndromes

In the treatment of a disease, TCM not only analyzes the disease but also the syndrome. The stress is on the analysis of the 'syndrome' first, and then the principle of the treatment is set up. For instance, the common cold, which is marked by fever and chills, headache and general aching. These symptoms suggest that the superficial part of the body has been affected. But a case of common cold may correspond to syndromes of either Wind Cold or Wind Heat, each linked to different pathogenic factors and body response. So only if a 'syndrome' of Wind Cold or Wind Heat type is determined, can herbal drugs either pungent warm in property or pungent cool in property be selected to relieve the exterior symptoms and signs and provide appropriate treatment of the common cold.

THE THEORIES OF YIN-YANG, AND THE FIVE ELEMENTS

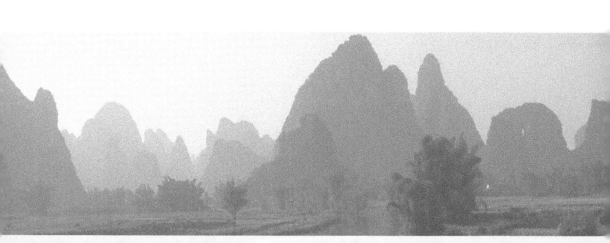

I. THE THEORY OF YIN-YANG

1. THE CONCEPT AND CHARACTERISTICS OF YIN AND YANG

1.1 Yin and Yang

Yin and Yang are general terms used to describe and encapsulate the opposite yet interdependent aspects of objects or natural phenomena. Together, they carry the meaning of opposition and unity. Yin and Yang may represent two opposing objects, such as Heaven and Earth, day and night, Water and Fire, brightness and dimness, etc.; or two opposite aspects of a single object, such as Qi and Blood, Zang and Fu, Yang meridians and Yin meridians of the body.

1.2 The original meaning and extended meaning

The original meaning of Yin and Yang refered to the sunny side and shady side, for example of a moutain. The side facing the sun is Yang; the side at the back, where the sun does not shine, Yin. Later, the meaning broadened to include all opposites. Yin and Yang were then used to denote cold and warm weather; downward or upward, left or right, exterior or interior direction; quiescence or dynamism concerning movement, etc.

2. YIN-YANG ATTRIBUTES

2.1 Attributes classified according to Yin-Yang

Generally speaking, things that are dynamic, external, ascending, warm, hot, or bright can be classified as Yang; things that are static, internal, descending, cold, cool, or dim can be classified as Yin. Chapter 5 of the book *Plain Questions* states: 'the left and right are the channels of Yin and Yang; Water and Fire are the symbols of Yin and Yang; Yin and Yang are the origin of birth.'

Attributes classified according to Yin–Yang

Yang	Yin
Dynamic	Static
External	Internal
Ascending	Descending
Warm	Cold
Bright	Dim
Nonsubstantial	Substantial
Functional	Material
Excitement	Inhibition
Promotion	Stagnation
Warming	Nourishing

2.2 Universality of Yin-Yang

All things or phenomena that have a relation to each other, or related aspects within the same object or phenomenon, can be classified and analyzed according to their Yin–Yang properties. It was pointed out in Chapter 5 of the book *Plain Questions*: 'Yin and Yang are the laws of heaven and Earth, the great framework of everything, the parents of change, the root and beginning of life and death, and the source of all mysteries.' In other words, everything that exists can be described in terms of Yin–Yang theory.

2.3 Relativity of Yin-Yang

The Yin or Yang nature of a phenomenon is not absolute but relative. Phenomena are Yin or Yang only in relation to other phenomena.

2.3.1 Infinite division of Yin-Yang

Yin and Yang are infinitely divisible. There is Yin–Yang within Yin and Yang. For instance, daytime pertains to Yang; night pertains to Yin. As far as the morning and afternoon of the day are concerned, the morning is Yang within Yang, afternoon is Yin within Yang as the day comes closer to night, and similarly; the first and second half of the night, the former is Yin within Yin, the latter Yang within Yin.

2.3.2 Mutual transformation of Yin-Yang

There is a dynamic mutual transforming relation between Yin and Yang. As circumstances change, Yin transforms into Yang and Yang transforms into Yin. Everything in the universe can be analyzed into Yin and Yang categories. Every object itself can be further divided into Yin and Yang aspects (the universality of Yin and Yang). Moreover, any aspect of Yin or Yang within a single object can be subdivided into Yin and Yang (the relativity of Yin and Yang). Countless phenomena in nature are opposite yet related to each other. As *Plain Questions* says, 'Yin and Yang could amount to ten in number; they could be extended to one hundred, one thousand, ten thousand or infinity; but although infinitely divisible, Yin and Yang are based upon only one important principle.'

3. THE BASIC NATURE OF YIN-YANG

3.1 Opposition of Yin-Yang

Yin and Yang are opposite in nature, yet control and restrain one another. The opposition of Yin and Yang is mainly manifested in their intercontrolling and consuming–supporting relationship. Only when Yin and Yang are not only in opposition, but also in unity, can a relative balance between Yin and Yang be maintained to ensure change and development in nature. If this balance is out of kilter, disease will be the result.

3.2 Inter-dependence between Yin and Yang

Yin and Yang are opposed to, and yet dependent on each other for existence. Neither Yin nor Yang can exist in isolation but only in relation to one another.

The interdependence between Yin and Yang reflects not only the relevant substantial and functional relations, but also the relation between substances and functions. If this relation of interdependence is out of balance, the body cannot perform its normal functions, resulting in disease.

3.3 Equilibrium of the mutual consuming-supporting relationship between Yin and Yang

The balance between Yin and Yang is neither fixed nor absolute. The relative equilibrium is maintained through their mutual consuming–supporting relation in which the consumption of Yin leads to the gaining of Yang, and the consumption of Yang leads to the gaining of Yin within certain limitations and over a period of time. The consuming–supporting relationship between Yin and Yang is absolute, while their balance is relative. Under conditions where the consuming–supporting relationship results in relative balance between Yin and Yang, normal life activities keep on going. If the consuming–supporting relationship exceeds normal physiological limits, then the relative balance of Yin and Yang will not be maintained, resulting in excess or deficiency of either Yin or Yang and therefore the occurrence of diseases.

4. APPLICATION OF THE THEORY OF YIN-YANG IN TCM

4.1 The organic structure of the human body

According to the properties of Yin and Yang, in terms of anatomical location, the upper part of the body is Yang and the lower part Yin; the exterior Yang and interior Yin; the lateral aspects of the limbs Yang and medial aspects Yin; the back Yang and abdomen Yin. As far as the Zang Fu organs are concerned, the five Zang organs pertain to Yin and the interior because they store Essence and don't excrete; the Fu organs pertain to Yang and the exterior because they transport and don't store. Within the five Zang organs, there are Yin and Yang aspects. The Heart and Lungs, situated in the upper part of the body (thorax), pertain to Yang, while the Liver, Spleen, and Kidneys, located in the lower part of the body (abdomen), pertain to Yin. Furthermore, within the specific organs, there are also Yin and Yang aspects, namely, Heart Yin, Heart Yang, etc.

4.2 The physiological functions of the human body

The normal vital activities of the human body are based on the coordination of Yin and Yang in a unity of opposites. Functional activities pertain to Yang, and nutrient substances pertain to Yin. The physiological activities of the body rely on the support of the nutrient substances. Without these substances, the body is unable to perform its functional activities; while at the same time, the physiological functional activities constantly promote the metabolism of the substances. The relationship between the functional activities and substances reflects the interdependent, interconsuming and supporting relationship between Yin and Yang. When Yin and Yang are no longer interdependent but separated, life reaches its end. Chapter 3 of *Plain Questions* says, 'When Yin is stabilized and Yang well-conserved, the spirit will be in harmony; separation of Yin and Yang results in exhaustion of essential Qi.'

4.3 Pathological changes of the human body

There should be a relative coordination between Yin and Yang in terms of the body structure, the internal and external, the upper and lower parts; the substances of the body, and the functions of the body whereby the interaction of the substances and functions of the body guarantee normal physiological activities. Yin and Yang are interdependent yet intercontrolled, consumed by each other and also supported. So, any disorder of Yin and Yang will cause either deficiency or excess of Yin or Yang, resulting in disease.

However, the occurrence and development of a disease is also related to the strength of the antipathogenic Qi and pathogenic factors. Antipathogenic Qi relates to the structure and functions of the whole body, including the body's resistance to diseases; pathogenic factors include all kinds of causative factors of disease.

Antipathogenic Qi consists of both Yin and Yang, including Yin fluid and Yang Qi. Equally, pathogenic factors can be distinguished as Yin or Yang pathogenic factors. For instance, among the six exogenous factors, Cold and Damp are Yin pathogenic factors; Wind, Summer Heat, Heat (Fire), Dryness are Yang pathogenic factors. The course of a disease is usually a process of the conflict between antipathogenic Qi and pathogenic factors, resulting in excess or deficiency of Yin and Yang. So, the pathogenic changes of diseases are no more than the conditions of excess or deficiency of Yin and Yang.

4.3.1 Excess of Yin-Yang

Excess of Yin or excess of Yang means a pathological condition in which Yin or Yang is excessive beyond the normal balanced level.

Excess of Yang leads to Heat, resulting in a Yin disease. Generally speaking, Yang excess syndromes are usually caused by Yang pathogenic factors in which Yang is absolutely excessive. When Yang increases, Yin decreases. So, excess of Yang will inevitably consume Yin, giving rise to a Yin disease.

Excess of Yin leads to Cold, resulting in a Yang disease. Yin excess syndromes are usually caused by Yin pathogenic factors in which Yin is absolutely excessive. When Yin increases, Yang decreases. So, excess of Yin will inevitably injure Yang, giving rise to a Yang disease.

4.3.2 Deficiency of Yin-Yang

Deficiency of Yin or Yang constitutes a pathological condition in which Yin or Yang is deficient in relation to the normal balance.

Yang deficiency leads to Cold, indicating weakened and consumed Yang Qi of the body. When Yang is deficient, it is unable to restrain Yin, resulting in Cold symptoms and signs caused by relative excess of Yin.

Yin deficiency leads to Heat, indicating lack of Yin fluid within the body. When Yin is deficient, it fails to control Yang, resulting in Heat symptoms and signs caused by relative excess of Yang.

Injured Yang affecting Yin: This is a phenomenon of Yang deficiency to the degree that there is failure to generate Yin fluid, leading to the simultaneous presence of Yin deficiency.

Injured Yin affecting Yang: This is a phenomenon of Yin deficiency to the degree that there is failure to promote Yang Qi, leading to the simultaneous presence of Yang deficiency.

Both Yin and Yang being affected: This develops from injured Yang affecting Yin and injured Yin affecting Yang, but does not mean that the balance between Yin and Yang is lost. Within the condition the difference between relative Yang deficiency or Yin deficiency still exists.

4.3.3 Transformation of Yin and Yang

A pathological condition caused by the imbalance of Yin and Yang may, under certain circumstances, transform into its opposite, i.e. a Yang syndrome may transform into Yin syndrome, or a Yin syndrome into a Yang syndrome. Such change may be discussed as 'extreme Cold brings about Heat, and extreme Heat causes Cold; extreme Yin gives rise to Yang and extreme Yang leads to Yin.'

4.4 Diagnosis of diseases

For the differentiation of syndromes, there are eight principles, namely, Yin, Yang, exterior, interior, Cold, Heat, deficiency and excess. But among the eight principles, Yin and Yang are the main and fundamental principles. The exterior, excess and Heat are generalized into Yang; while the interior, deficiency and Cold into Yin. In clinical practice, when making syndrome differentiation, Yin and Yang should be determined first, in order to grasp the nature of the disease, following the principle of determining the simple in order to deal with the complicated. In general, a syndrome may be attributed to either Yin or Yang, and, in more precise analysis, a particular pulse also can be attributed to Yin or Yang.

4.5 Treatment of diseases

The root cause of the occurrence and development of a disease is the imbalance between Yin and Yang. So, the basic treatment principle is to regulate and adjust Yin–Yang, to reduce the excess, support the deficiency and restore the relative balance between Yin and Yang.

4.5.1 Setting up principles of treatment

Principles of treatment for Yin or Yang excess – reducing the excess: The principle of reducing the excess is used to treat either a Yin excess or Yang excess syndrome in which the opposite side has not yet been deficient and weakened. Yang excess syndrome, a Heat syndrome of excess type, should be treated with drugs that are Cold and cool in nature in order to restrain Yang. This conforms to the principle of 'treating Heat by Cold'. Yin excess syndrome, a Cold syndrome of excess type, should be treated with drugs that are warm and hot in nature in order to restrain Yin. And this conforms to the principle of 'treating Cold by Heat'.

Principles of treatment for Yin or Yang deficiency: When Yin is deficient, it fails to restrain Yang, giving rise to hyperactivity of Yang, resulting in a Heat syndrome of the deficient type. In such cases, Heat should not be reduced directly by using drugs that are Cold in nature. Instead, a method of 'nourishing Yin and replenishing fluid for control of Yang' can be applied to tonify Yin and check hyperactive Yang. This principle is called 'treating Yin for a Yang disease' in *Internal Classic*.

Equally, when Yang is deficient, it fails to restrain Yin, leading to excess of Yin, and therefore a Cold syndrome of the deficient type. In treating a Cold deficient syndrome, drugs that are pungent and warm in nature and used for dispersing Yin Cold are not appropriate. Instead, the principle of treatment should be based on strengthening Yang to cause excessive Yin to retreat. This is known as 'treating Yang for a Yin disease' in *Internal Classic*.

In the treatment of deficiency of Yin or Yang, the physician Zhang Jingyue put forward the principle of gaining Yang from Yin and gaining Yin from Yang, based on the interdependence of Yin and Yang. This principle explains that 'those who know how to tonify Yang are able to obtain Yang from Yin, because gaining Yang promotes Yin for further production and transformation; those who know how to tonify Yin are able to obtain Yin from Yang, because gaining Yin strengthens Yang for constant generation of Water and Fluid.'

To sum up, the basic principle of treatment is to reduce excess and reinforce deficiency so as to treat abnormal conditions of excess or deficiency of either Yin or Yang and restore the relative balance between them.

4.5.2 Summarizing the actions of drugs

The actions of a drug usually depend on its Qi (nature), taste, and directions of ascending, descending, floating or sinking, which can all be summarized by Yin and Yang.

Nature of drug: There are four types of nature: Cold, Hot, Warm and Cool, namely, 'four Qi', among which the Cold and Cool natures pertain to Yin, and the Warm and Hot natures pertain to Yang. The drugs that can clear Heat to relieve Heat symptoms and signs pertain to a Cold or Cool nature, such as Huangqin (黄芩*Radix Scutellariae*), Zhizi (栀子 *Pructus Gardeniae*), etc. The drugs that can dispel Cold to relieve Cold symptoms and signs pertain to a Warm or Hot nature, such as Fuzi (附子 *Radix Aconiti Praeparata*), Ganjiang (干姜 *Rhizoma Zingiberis*), etc.

Five tastes: There are five fundamental tastes: pungent, sweet, sour, bitter and salty. Some drugs have a tasteless taste or a mouth-puckering taste. Among them, pungent, sweet, tasteless tastes pertain to Yang, while sour, bitter, salty tastes pertain to Yin.

Ascending, descending, floating and sinking: This refers to the ascending, descending, floating–dispersing, and sedative functions of drugs. The drugs with ascending, floating–dispersing functions pertain to Yang and can lift Yang and disperse the exterior, dispel Wind and Cold, cause vomiting, and open the orifice for resuscitation. And drugs marked by descending–sinking features pertain to Yin. These often have purgative, Heat-reducing, urine-promoting, sedative, digestion-promoting and astringent effects.

II. THE THEORY OF THE FIVE ELEMENTS

1. THE BASIC CONCEPT OF THE FIVE ELEMENTS (WU XING)

Wood, Fire, Earth, Metal and Water are the five basic elements based on which the movement and changes of all things in nature can be classified into five categories. 'Wu' refers to the five basic substances, namely Wood, Fire, Earth, Metal and Water; 'Xing' has two meanings: ranks, order; and movement and changes.

2. THE NATURE OF THE FIVE ELEMENTS

2.1 Characteristics of the Five Elements

The fundamental laws to analyze the classification of things and phenomena, as well as their interrelations according to the Five Elements, though abstract, were summarized and developed gradually. They were based on the ancient Chinese people's naive way of thinking through their objective observation in nature of Wood, Fire, Earth, Metal and Water in their daily life and working experience.

The characteristics of the Five Elements can be summarized as 'Water, moistening; Fire, flaring up; Wood, straight growing; Metal, transforming; Earth, sowing and crops growing.'

2.1.1 Characteristics of Water

'Water moistens and flows downward.' Anything that is cold, cool in nature, moistens, and flows downward corresponds to Water.

2.1.2 Characteristics of Fire

'Fire flares up.' It is warm and hot in nature. Anything that is warm, hot, and rising corresponds to Fire.

2.1.3 Characteristics of Wood

'Wood grows straight.' Having a germination process, it spreads out freely. Its extended meanings include growing, ascending, flourishing and being harmonious. Things marked by these properties can be classified into the category of Wood.

2.1.4 Characteristics of Metal

'Metal causes transformation and change.' The characteristic of Metal is to descend and be clear with astringent effect. Things with the nature of Metal are classified into Metal category.

2.1.5 Characteristics of Earth

'Earth gives birth to all things.' It serves in sowing and the growth of crops. It represents germination and production, and is marked by receiving and nurturing features. So, 'Earth is the mother of all things.' Those things with the characteristics of Earth are classified into Earth category.

2.2 Five categories of things classified according to the Five Elements

Concrete objects or phenomena are compared to the properties of the Five Elements by analogy. Anything that displays these properties will be classified into the category of the related element.

Five Elements Correspondences

	Nature							Human body						
Notes	Tastes	Colours	Changes	Climate	Direction	Seasons	Five Elements	Five Zang	Six Fu	Senses	Tissues	Emotion	Voice	Action
Jiao	Sour	Green	Germinate	Wind	East	Spring	Wood	Liver (LR)	Gallbladder (GB)	Eye	Tendon	Anger	Shout	Grip
Zhi	Bitter	Red	Grow	Heat	South	Summer	Fire	Heart (HT)	Small Intestine (SI)	Tongue	Vessel	Joy	Laugh	Restlessness
Gong	Sweet	Yellow	Transform	Damp	Middle	Late summer	Earth	Spleen (SP)	Stomach (ST)	Mouth	Muscle	Over-thinking	Sing	Vomit
Shang	Pungent	White	Reap	Dryness	West	Autumn	Metal	Lungs (LU)	Large Intestine (LI)	Nose	Skin, hair	Grief	Cry	Cough
Yu	Salty	Black	Store	Cold	North	Winter	Water	Kidneys (KI)	Bladder (BL)	Ear	Bone	Fear	Groan	Shiver

2.2.1 Finding similes by analogy

Finding similes by analogy involves comparing the properties and functions of objects and phenomena to those of the Five Elements so as to discover the attributes of the Five Elements. For example, the following are directions attributed to the Five Elements:

- Since the sun rises in the East, the rising of the sun is similar to the upward growth of trees, so the East is classified into the Wood category.

- The weather in the South is hot, similar to the warm and upward flaring property of Fire, thus, the South is classified into the Fire category.

- The sun sets in the West, and the sun setting is similar to the descending property of Metal, so the West is classified into the Metal category.

- The weather in the North is cold, similar to the cold property of Water, thus the North is classified into the Water category.

2.2.2 Classification by inference

Classification by inference involves classifying other related things and phenomena according to the known attributes of the Five Elements. According to TCM theory:

- The Liver pertains to Wood; its meridian connects with the Gallbladder with which it is internally–externally related. It controls the tendons, opens into the eye and has its manifestation in the nails. Therefore, the Gallbladder, tendons, and eyes, which are related to the Liver, are all classified into the Wood category.

- The Spleen pertains to Earth; physiologically it is related to the following aspects: the internal–external relationship between the Spleen and Stomach; dominating the muscles, opening into the mouth and manifesting on the lips. So, the Stomach, muscles, mouth and lips are also classified into the Earth category.

2.3 Inter-promoting, interacting, overacting and counteracting relationships among the Five Elements

The Theory of the Five Elements explores and explains the relationship between the internal related parts and mechanism of the self-adjustment of the complex system within the laws of interpromotion and interaction. These laws reflect the unification and integration, as well as the influences caused by the breakdown of the equilibrium as a result of overacting and counteracting relationships (see Figure 1.1).

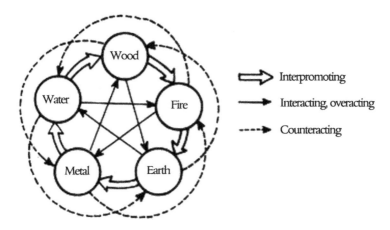

Figure 1.1: The relationships between the Five Elements

2.3.1 Interpromoting or generating relationship among the Five Elements

Interpromotion refers to mutual production and generation, whereby each Element gives birth to one of the others.

The order of interpromotion is: Wood promotes Fire; Fire promotes Earth; Earth promotes Metal; Metal promotes Water; Water promotes Wood.

2.3.2 The controlling relationship among the Five Elements

Interacting here means to bring under control.

The order of interaction is: Wood acts on Earth; Earth acts on Water; Water acts on Fire, Fire acts on Metal; Metal acts on Wood.

The generating and controlling relationships among the Five Elements are normal phenomena in nature as well as normal physiological phenomena of the body. Because of such relationships, ecological equilibrium in nature and physiological balance in the human body are maintained. So, 'promotion is based on restriction'. Since there exist interpromoting and interacting relationships among the Five Elements, each of the Five Elements both promotes and is promoted; it acts on one of the other, and is at the same time acted upon by one of the other elements.

The 'being promoted' and 'promoting' relationship was called the 'mother' and 'child' relationship in *Classic on Medical Problems*. The one that promotes is the 'mother', and the one being promoted is the 'child'. So, the interpromoting relationship among the Five Elements is also known as the 'mother and child' relationship. Take Fire, for example: Wood promotes Fire and Fire promotes Earth; Wood is the 'mother' of Fire, Earth is the 'child' of Fire. In this sense, Wood and Fire have the 'mother–child' relationship, as do Fire and Earth.

The interacting or controlling relationship was known as 'the acted upon (controlled)' and 'acting upon (controlling)' relationship in *Internal Classic*. Take Fire, for example: Fire acts on Metal, Metal is the 'acted upon' element. Water acts on Fire, so it is the 'acting upon' element.

2.3.3 Interaction of the Five Elements

The interpromotion and interaction relationships coexist and are mutually connected, and this maintains the coordination and balance among the Five Elements.

2.3.4 Overaction (overcontrol) of the Five Elements

Either overstrength of the acting part or overweakness of the part acted upon can result in the acting abnormality.

The sequence of overaction (which is the same as that of interaction) is: Wood overacts on Earth; Earth on Water; Water on Fire; Fire on Metal; Metal on Wood.

The reasons for overaction involve the following two aspects:

1. One Element of the five is overstrong itself, leading to excessive control of the controlled Element, which induces the weakness of the controlled Element, resulting in an abnormality of promotion and restriction among the Five Elements. For instance, the overstrength of Wood results in overacting on Earth, thus an insufficiency of Earth results, described as 'Wood overacts on Earth.'

2. If one Element of the five is itself weak, in corresponding to its normal controlling Element, the interaction will seem to be stronger, thus this Element will be even weaker. For instance, Wood itself is not strong enough in itself to overcontrol, and its acting on Earth may be still within normal limits. But if Earth itself is insufficient, the interaction between Wood and Earth will become relatively strong, leading to even more insufficiency of Earth, termed as 'Wood overacts on Earth when Earth is deficient.'

2.3.5 Counteraction (countercontrol) of the Five Elements

One element of the Five counteracts on its controlling Element.

The sequence of counteraction is: Wood counteracts on Metal, Metal on Fire, Fire on Water, Water on Earth, Earth on Wood.

For instance, Wood should be controlled by Metal. If Wood is especially strong, it will be not only fail to be controlled by Metal, but, on the contrary, it counteracts on Metal; this is termed 'Wood counteracts on Metal.' If Metal is quite weak, it will not only fail to control Wood, but will be counteracted by Wood, which is described as 'Metal is counteracted by Wood when it is weak.'

Interaction, overaction and counteraction of the Five Elements is shown in Figure 1.2.

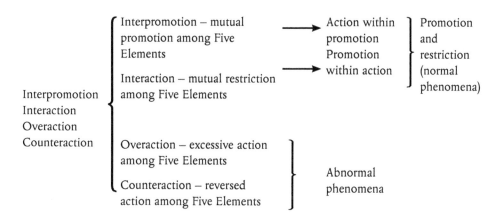

Figure 1.2: Interaction, overaction and counteraction of the Five Elements

2.3.6 Differences and relationships between overaction (overcontrol) and counteraction

Differences: Overaction manifests the excessive action as part of the sequence of interaction among the Five Elements and represents an abnormality in the actions of promotion and restriction among the Five Elements. Counteraction presents the restriction in the form of a reversed sequence of interaction among the Five Elements and also represents an abnormality in the actions of promotion and restriction among the Five Elements.

Relationships: Counteraction may happen at the same time when overcontrol presents, and vice versa. For example, if Wood is over-strong, it may not only over-act on Earth, but also counteract on Metal. If Metal is deficient, it may not only be counteracted by Wood, but also be overcontrolled by Fire.

3. APPLICATION OF THE FIVE ELEMENTS IN CHINESE MEDICINE

The Five Elements are not only essential to the theoretic explanation of Chinese medicine, but are also of practical significance in clinical guidance.

3.1 To explain the physiologic functions of the five Zang organs* and their interrelationships

The Theory of the Five Elements classifies the internal organs of the human body into five categories and explains the physiologic functions of the five Zang organs in terms of the characteristics of the Five Elements. For example, Wood is characterized as free in flexion and extension, as the branches and leaves of a tree are free, movable and growing in property. Liver prefers free movement and dislikes being prohibited, and it functions to promote the free flow of Qi. Thus, Liver pertains to Wood.

The physiologic applications of the Five Elements are outlined below.

3.1.1

The five Zang organs correspond to the Five Elements and also connect with their own five tissues, five organs, five mental states, etc. Hence, every part of the body is connected organically, and the physiopathologic system is formed, in which the five Zang organs are the core – all of which expresses the holistic nature of the human body.

3.1.2

In the light of the law of promotion and control cycle, Five Elements theory explains the interconnection and intercontrol among the five systems in the body, namely the Liver, Heart, Spleen, Lungs and Kidneys, and further establishes a complete organic, holistic, fundamental idea of the human body.

3.1.3

The classification in terms of the Five Elements in which the five Zang organs are taken as the core explains the unity within the mutual connection between the human body and its external environment.

3.2 To explain the mutual influences on the disorders of the five Zang organs

The five Zang organs have a mutual impact on one another pathologically. The disorder of one organ may transfer to another, and vice versa. Such mutual impact is termed 'transmission'. The transmission in interpromotion includes sickness of the mother organ transferring into the son organ, and vice versa. The transmission in terms of interaction includes overcontrol and counteraction.

---

*   For a full explanation of the Zang and Fu organs, see Chapter 2.

3.3 To guide diagnosis and treatment

The five Zang organs, five colours, five tones and five flavours of the human body are all classified through the Five Elements. In clinical diagnosis of disease, the nature of the disease is deduced in the context of the relevant classification and the laws of interpromotion, interaction, overcontrol and counteraction on the basis of the information collected by inspection, auscultation and olfaction, inquiry and palpation.

3.3.1 To determine the principle of treatment in terms of the law of interpromotion: tonify mother for deficiency, reduce child for excess

The common methods of treatment are as follows:

Nourish Water to replenish Wood: Nourish Kidney Yin to replenish Liver Yin, indicated by insufficiency of Liver Yin and hyperactivity of Liver Yang due to Kidney deficiency.

Cultivate Earth to produce Metal: Tonify Spleen-Qi to benefit Lung-Qi, indicated by deficiency of the Lungs and Spleen due to weakness of the Spleen and the Stomach resulting in their failing to nourish the Lungs.

Mutual-production of Metal and Water: This is a method used to nourish Lung and Kidney Yin in deficiency syndrome, indicated by Yin deficiency of the Lungs and Kidneys due to Lung deficiency failing to nourish the Kidneys.

3.3.2 To determine suppression or enhancement in terms of the law of overcontrol

The common methods of treatment are as follows:

Suppress Wood and support Earth: This is a method used for Liver excess and Spleen deficiency in which drugs are used for soothing the Liver and strengthening the Spleen, indicated by the syndrome induced by Wood hyperactivity overacting on Earth, and Wood failing to regulate Earth.

Cultivate Earth and administer Water: This is the method used for retention of harmful fluids and Damp by the use of drugs for warming Spleen Yang or warming the Kidneys and strengthening the Spleen, indicated by oedema, fullness and distention caused by Spleen deficiency failing in its work of transportation.

Assist Metal and suppress Wood: This is a method used for suppressing Liver Wood so as to allow Lung-Qi to descend, indicated by the syndrome induced by hyperactive Liver Fire preventing Lung-Qi from descending.

Reduce South and replenish North: This means reducing Heart Fire and nourishing Kidney Water, indicated by insufficiency of Kidney Yin, hyperactivity of Heart Fire, disharmony of Water and Fire and disharmony of Heart and Kidney.

3.3.3 To guide psychotherapy in terms of the Theory of the Five Elements

Emotions are generated from the five Zang organs. Hence the relationships of interpromotion and interaction among the five Zang organs extend to the emotions.

- **Grief** is from the Lungs and pertains to Metal; anger is from the Liver and pertains to Wood. Metal acts on Wood, hence, grief conquers anger.

- **Fear** is from the Kidneys and pertains to Water; joy is from the Heart and pertains to Fire. Water acts on Fire, hence, fear conquers joy.

- **Anger** is from the Liver and pertains to Wood; thinking is from the Spleen and pertains to Earth. Wood acts on Earth, hence, anger conquers thinking.

- **Joy** is from the Heart and pertains to Fire; grief is from the Lungs and pertains to Metal. Fire acts on Metal, hence, joy conquers grief.

- **Thinking** is from the Spleen and pertains to Earth; fear is from the Kidneys and pertains to Water. Earth acts on Water, hence, thinking conquers fear.

CHAPTER 2

THE THEORY OF THE
ZANG FU ORGANS

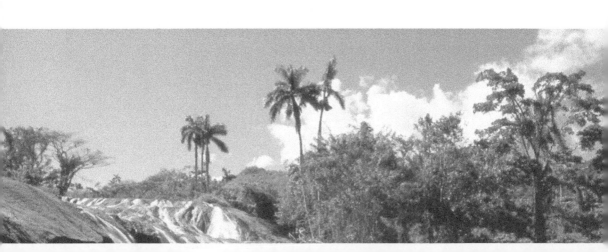

I. BRIEF INTRODUCTION

There are five Zang organs (which are Yin in nature), and six Fu organs (Yang in nature). In addition, there are six Extraordinary Fu organs.

The Zang and Fu organs and the Extraordinary Fu organs

	Zang organs	Fu organs	Extraordinary Fu organs
Nature	Yin	Yang	
Number	5	6	6
	Heart	Small Intestine	Brain
	Lungs	Large Intestine	Marrow
	Spleen	Stomach	Bones
	Liver	Gallbladder	Vessels
	Kidneys	Bladder	Gallbladder
		Triple Burner	Uterus

1. THE BASIC CONCEPTS OF ZANG XIANG THEORY

Zang: Internal organs stored in the interior of the body.

Xiang: Physio-pathological phenomena manifested on the exterior of the body.

Zang Xiang theory: The study of the physiological function, pathological changes and the interrelationships of the internal organs in the human body through the observation of human physiopathological conditions.

2. COMMON PHYSIOLOGICAL CHARACTERISTICS OF ZANG XIANG

Plain Questions says: 'the five Zang organs mainly have the function of storing Essence, hence they are full of Essence but not food; and the six Fu organs mainly have the function of transmitting and transforming food and water, hence they are full of foodstuff but not Essence.' The five Zang organs, six Fu organs and the Extraordinary organs are classified in terms of physiological characteristics.

Common physiological characteristics of the five Zang organs: To produce and preserve essential Qi.

Common physiological characteristics of the six Fu organs: To receive, digest Water and food and to excrete the waste products.

Common physiological characteristics of the Extraordinary Fu organs: The physiological functions of the organs in this category are different from those of the six Fu organs. They have no direct contact with water and food, but they are the relatively closed tissues and organs. In addition, they have a similar function to the Zang organs in preserving essential Qi.

The differences between the Zang, Fu and extraordinary Fu organs are outlined below.

	Function	Morphology	Characteristics	Relationship with meridian
Five Zang	Produce and preserve essential Qi	Solid organs	Storage without excretion, full of Essence without foodstuff	Be related, dominate the interior and pertain to Yin
Six Fu	Transmit and digest water and food	Hollow cavity	Excretion without storage, full of foodstuff without Essence	Be related, dominate the exterior and pertain to Yang
Extraordinary Fu	Store essential Qi	Hollow cavity	Same as those of five Zang organs (except the Gallbladder)	No relationship (except the Gallbladder)

3. THE FORMATION OF ZANG XIANG THEORY

3.1 Ancient recognition of anatomy
Classic of Internal Medicine has described in detail the human structure, in which lies the morphologic basis of the formation of Zang Xiang theory

3.2 Long-term observation of life practice

By the holistic observation of human life phenomena
By the analysis on interrelationships of phenomena
} Understand step by step the laws of physiopathology changes

Knowing the interior by observing the exterior
Analogy
Holistic observation
Generalization
by the analysis of interrelationships of phenomena and abstract inference and induction

3.3 Penetration of ancient philosophical thoughts

Theory of essential Qi
Theory of Yin–Yang
Theory of Five Elements
} Penetrate Chinese medicine theories, which played an important role in the formation and systematization of Zang Xiang theory and enabled the Zang Fu conception to evolve from morphological substance to a functional model

3.4 Accumulated experience of medical practice
Understanding the interrelationships of organs and tissues by analysis and repeated validations of therapeutic effects

Figure 2.1: The formation of Zang Xiang theory

4. THE MAIN CHARACTERISTICS OF ZANG XIANG THEORY

By this we mean the holistic idea that takes the five Zang organs as the core, embodied as follows.

Yin and Yang division based on the Zang Fu organs: One Yin and one Yang organ are related externally and internally. Zang and Fu together make a whole. For instance, the Heart is related externally and internally to the Small Intestine, the Lungs to the Large Intestine, the Spleen to the Stomach, the Liver to the Gallbladder, the Kidneys to the Bladder and the Pericardium to the Triple Burner.

The external–internal relationship of the Zang Fu organs is mainly in terms of the running courses of the meridians that are paired as Yin and Yang and inter-connected with the collaterals. Each Zang organ is closely connected with a Fu organ in physiology.

The five Zang organs connect with tissues and orifices and they have specific connections with each of the outward manifestations and orifices: In terms of Zang Xiang theory, the Heart is manifested outward on the face, dominates Blood and vessel and opens into the tongue; the Lungs are manifested outward in the body hair, dominate the skin and open into the nose; the Spleen is manifested outward in the lips, dominates muscles and opens into the mouth; the Liver is manifested outward in the nails, dominates tendons and opens into the eyes; the Kidneys are manifested outward in the hair, dominate bone and open into the ears, and relate to urination and defecation.

Physiological activity of five Zang organs is closely related to the spirits and emotions: Spiritual emotions and consciousness activity in a human are the function of the brain. But in terms of Zang Xiang theory, it is understood that spiritual emotions and conscious activity tightly connect with the physiological activity of the five Zang organs. The dysfunction of the five Zang organs impacts on the spiritual emotions and consciousness activity of the brain, and vice versa.

Balancing coordination among the physiological functions of the five Zang organs is the critical step in maintaining the equilibrium of the internal environment: The balancing coordination of the internal environment of the human body is maintained through the relationships between the five Zang organs and the tissues and orifices, the connection between the five Zang organs and spiritual emotions and the communication between internal and external environments in the body.

The unity between the five Zang organs and the natural environment: There is not only the unity in the human body itself but also the harmony between the human body and natural environment. The functions of the five Zang organs are closely related to seasonal climatic changes. For example, the Liver functions are more hyperactive in spring, so people are more likely to have Liver diseases. In autumn, there will be more diseases of the Lung when it is dry and the Lung is affected. In addition, different geographical conditions, food, housing and living habits can all influence the functions of the five Zang organs, bringing about different constitution and diseases.

5. DIFFERENCES BETWEEN 'ZANG FU' ORGANS AND 'VISCERAL' ORGANS

The differences between a 'Zang Fu' and a 'visceral' organ are shown in Figure 2.2.

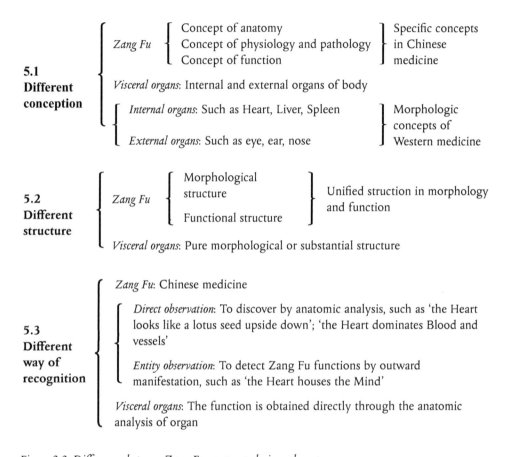

Figure 2.2: Differences between Zang Fu organs and visceral organs

II. THE FIVE ZANG ORGANS

Five Zang organs is the general term for the Heart, Lungs, Spleen, Liver and Kidneys. The main physiological functions and specialisms of the five Zang organs are outlined below.

1. THE HEART

Of the Five Elements, the Heart belongs to Fire in Five Elements theory, dominates vital activity and is the monarch organ. The Heart opens into the tongue and is manifested outward in the complexion; it is related to joy and its fluid is sweat. The Heart is related to the Small Intestine externally and internally.

The main physiological functions of the Heart are listed below.

1.1 Controlling Blood and blood vessels

Blood and blood vessels are involved in this function. Blood runs throughout the whole body in blood vessels and is transported to the whole body by means of the Heart beating and bringing its nourishment into play. A vessel is the holder of Blood and is the pathway of Blood circulation. Whether or not the vessel pathway is smooth, and whether or not the functions of nutrient Qi and Blood are sound, may directly affect the normal circulation of Blood. The physiological function of this system is governed by the Heart and relies on the normal beating of the Heart. The normal Heart beat is viewed as relying on Heart-Qi in terms of the theory of Chinese medicine. Only if the Heart-Qi is abundant, can Heart strength be normal, Heart rate and Heart rhythm be maintained and Blood run constantly and normally in the vessels in order to provide nutrients to the whole body.

The necessary conditions for good Blood circulation in vessels are: abundant Heart-Qi and abundant Blood and sound circulation in the bood vessel pathways (see Figure 2.3). Abundant Heart-Qi is manifested in a red and lustrous complexion, and a moderate and forceful pulse. Insufficiency of Heart-Qi, deficiency of Blood and poor circulation in vessels may present as a lustreless complexion, and a thready and weak pulse. Even worse, Qi and Blood stagnation and obstruction of blood vessels may present as a dark complexion, with cyanosis of the lips, a purplish tongue, precordial distress and pricking pain, as well as a knotted pulse, intermittent pulse, hesitant pulse, abrupt pulse, etc.

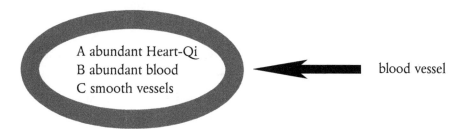

Figure 2.3: Necessary conditions for good Blood circulation

1.2 Taking charge of mental activities

The ability to take charge of mental activities is also known as 'the Heart housing the Mind (Shen)'. 'Shen' can be understood in a broad or narrow sense.

- *Broad sense:* This refers to the validities – the external appearances of the life activities of the human body as a whole, such as the whole image of the person, the eye expression, speech, physical and verbal responses, body movements and postures.

- *Narrow sense:* This refers to the Mind housed in the Heart, where it refer to the workings of the Mind, consciousness and the thoughts of the human body. *Miraculous Pivot* says 'the Heart functions by receiving information from the exterior'.

The normal physiological function of the Heart in taking charge of mental activities provides vigorous spirits, clear consciousness, keen thoughts and alert responses to external information. If dysfunctional, it may present as insomnia, dreamdisturbed sleep, restlessness, even delirium and mania, or present as a dull response, poor memory, low spirits, even coma or loss of consciousness in the clinic.

The relationship between controlling Blood and vessels and taking charge of mental activities

The mentality, consciousness and thoughts of the human body refer to the physiological function of the brain, meaning the response of the brain to external objects. In the Zang Xiang theory of Chinese medicine, the mentality, consciousness and thoughts not only belong to the five Zang organs, but also to the physiological functions of the Heart. The physiological function of the Heart in taking charge of mental activities is closely related to that of the Heart in controlling Blood and vessels. Blood is the substance that is the foundation of mental activities. The physiological function of the Heart in controlling Blood and vessels bring with it the function of taking charge of mental activity. Hence, any dysfunction of the Heart in controlling Blood and vessels must present as mental alterations.

1.3 The Heart as related to emotion, fluid, tissue and orifice

1.3.1 The Heart being related to joy

The physiological function of the Heart is related to joy. Generally speaking, if the Heart takes excessive charge of mental activities, it will cause uncontrollable laughing. However, a Heart deficiency in taking charge of mental activities will make a person susceptible to grief. Because the Heart controls the spirits and Mind, excessive joy as well as other excessive emotional states can impair the Heart-Mind, the Mind housed in the Heart.

1.3.2 Sweat as the fluid of the Heart

Yang Qi transforms Body Fluid into sweat through steaming and Qi activity, which is then secreted from the sweat glands. The secretion of sweat depends on the function of Wei Qi (defensive Qi) in controlling the opening and closing of the pores of the skin. The opening of the pores results in sweating and the closing in anhidrosis. Sweat is transformed from Body Fluid, and Blood and Body Fluid have the same source. Therefore, it follows that 'sweat and Blood share the same source'. Blood is controlled by the Heart; hence sweat is the Fluid of the Heart.

1.3.3 The Heart being associated with the bood vessels and having its outward manifestations in the face

The Heart being associated with the bood vessels means that the Blood and vessels of the entire body belong to the Heart. Having its outward manifestations in the face means that whether or not the physiological functions of the Heart are normal can be reflected in changes in the colour of the face. The face is rich in Blood and blood vessels. When Heart-Qi is sufficient and Blood is plentiful, the face will appear red and the skin moist. When Heart-Qi is insufficient, the face will appear pale, dark and gloomy. Blood deficiency results in a lustreless complexion and Blood stagnation develops as a cyanotic complexion.

1.3.4 The Heart having its special orifice in the tongue

The tongue is the outward manifestation of the Heart, and is referred to as the 'seedling of the Heart'. The tongue takes charge of the sense of taste and speech. Its functioning in taking charge of the sense of taste and correct language expression relies on the physiological functions of the Heart in controlling Blood and bood vessels and taking charge of mental activity. If the physiological functions of the Heart are abnormal, changes in the sense of taste, tongue rigidity, and delirium are induced.

1.4 The Pericardium

This is also called 'Tan Zhong'. It is the peripheral tissue of the Heart and has the function of protecting the Heart.

2. THE LUNGS

In terms of Five Elements theory, the Lungs belong to Metal and are located in the highest position and termed 'canopy'. The pulmonary lobe is delicate, unable to tolerate Cold and Heat and susceptible to attack by pathogenic factors; hence it is named the 'delicate organ'. The Lungs assist the Heart in regulating Qi and Blood circulation and hold 'the office of prime minister and instructor'. The Lungs open into the nose, are associated with the skin and have their outward manifestation in body hair. The Lungs are related to melancholy and their Fluid is nasal mucus. The Lungs are related to the Large Intestine externally and internally.

The main physiological functions of the Lungs are as follows.

2.1 Taking charge of Qi and respiration

The Lungs oversee the operation of the Qi of the whole body and take charge of respiration (see Figure 2.4).

Overseeing the Qi of the whole body: First, regarding the formation of Qi, the Lungs play a special role in forming 'Zong Qi' (pectoral Qi) in particular. Zong Qi is a mixture of fresh air inhaled by the Lungs and food Essence that has been transformed and transported by the Spleen and Stomach. Second, the Lungs also regulate the Qi activity of the whole body, meaning the respiratory movement of the Lungs, described as the ascending, descending, entering and exiting of Qi. The rhythmic inhaling and exhaling of the Lungs play an important role in regulating the ascending, descending, entering and exiting of Qi in the whole body.

Taking charge of respiration: The Lungs are the organs that exchange gases between the interior and exterior of the body. The human body takes in fresh air and expels waste gas via the Lungs' respiratory function. In doing so, the Lungs promote the formation of Qi and regulate the ascending, descending, entering and exiting of Qi, thus ensuring the continuous operation of normal body metabolism.

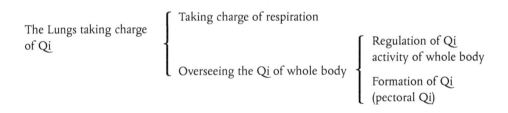

Figure 2.4: Taking charge of Qi

Even and rhythmic respiration of the Lungs is the fundamental condition of Qi formation and regular Qi activities. Respiratory dysfunction of the Lungs must impact on the formation of Zong Qi and Qi activities, and the Lungs' function is weakened in taking charge of Qi and respiration. If the Lungs loses their function in dominating respiration, vital activity will end. Hence, the Lungs' function in overseeing the Qi of the whole body chiefly relies on its function in taking charge of respiration. But Qi insufficiency, abnormal movements of ascending, descending, exiting and entering Qi, as well as abnormalities of Blood circulation, distribution and excretion of Body Fluids, may all affect the respiration of the Lungs and cause abnormal respiration to occur.

2.2 Taking charge of dispersing and descending

Dispersing function: This refers to the ascending of Lung-Qi and its disseminating throughout the body.

Descending: This refers to the sending down of Lung-Qi and clearing the respiratory tract.

2.2.1 There are three aspects of the dispersing physiological function of the Lungs

1. Expelling waste gas out of the body through the Qi activity of the Lungs.

2. Disseminating Body Fluid and food Essence transported to the Lungs by the Spleen throughout the whole body and externally to the skin and body hair.

3. Dispersing Wei Qi (defensive Qi), regulating the opening and closing of the skin pores and thereby discharging the sweat that has been transformed from Body Fluid after metabolism.

In pathology, if the Lungs develop a dysfunction in dispersing, dyspnoea, chest distress, asthma, cough, nasal obstruction, sneezing and anhidrosis can occur.

2.2.2 There are three aspects of the descending physiological function

1. Inhaling fresh air from the natural environment.

2. Sending down the fresh air, Body Fluid, and food Essence transported to the Lungs by the Spleen.

3. Clearing away foreign matter in the respiratory tract in order to keep the respiratory tract clean.

In pathology, if the Lungs develop an impairment of the normal functions of clarifying and sending down Lung-Qi, shortness of breath, shallow breathing, productive cough and haemoptysis can occur.

The relationship between dispersing and descending of the Lungs: The two functions are opposing, yet also complementary and inter-restraining. They are interdependent on each other in physiology and influence each other in pathology. Normal dispersing and descending result in a smooth respiratory tract, even breathing and normal gas exchange. A lack of coordination in dispersing and descending will result in 'sluggishness of Lung-Qi' and 'impairment of the normal clarifying and sending down of Lung-Qi'. This will lead to a cough and asthma.

2.3 Dredging and regulating the water passages

Water passages are the pathways for the movement and excretion of water. The Lungs' function in dredging and regulating the water passages refers to the role that the Lungs' dispersing and descending function plays in the dissemination, movement and excretion of water in the body. The Lungs' dispersing function disseminates Body Fluid and food Essence throughout the body, dominates the opening and closing of the skin pores and regulates the excretion of sweat. The Lungs' descending function sends the fresh Qi inhaled down to the Kidneys, transports water in the body constantly downward to become the source of urine. Through the Qi activities of the Kidneys and Bladder, the urine is formed and excreted. Hence it states 'the Lungs help maintain normal water metabolism' and 'the Lungs are the upper source of water circulation'.

In pathology, a dysfunction in the Lungs' dispersing function may impact on its function in dredging and regulating the water passages. An impairment of the normal function of clarifying and sending down Lung-Qi may lead to the failure of water being disseminated to the skin and body hair or failure in the opening and closing of the skin pores, and thus anhidrosis, or even oedema, may occur. A dysfunction in descending results in the failure of water to be transported to the Bladder, which leads to dysuria and oedema.

The process of water metabolism is illustrated in Figure 2.5.

2.4 Converging the bood vessels and governing the coordinating activities of the viscera

Converging of vessels: The Blood from the whole body converges in the Lungs through bood vessels and here the Lungs' respiratory function exchanges waste gas for fresh air, and then the Blood is disseminated to all parts of the body.

Governing the coordinating activities of the viscera: The Lungs are responsible for the coordination of visceral activities, including four main aspects:

1. Taking charge of respiration, which is rhythmical.

2. Operating and regulating Qi movement throughout the body associated with the Lungs' breathing, i.e. the ascending, descending, exiting and entering of Qi.

3. Assisting the Heart to propel Blood and regulate Blood circulation via the regulation of Qi activity.

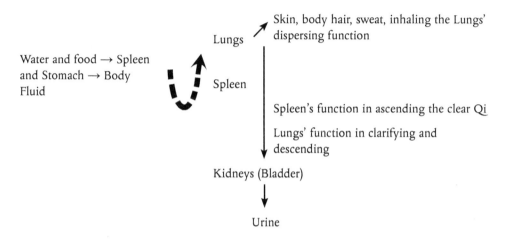

Figure 2.5: The process of the metabolism of water

4. The Lungs' dispersing and descending functions, which dominate and regulate the dissemination, circulation and excretion of Body Fluid.

2.5 The Lungs' relation to melancholy; nasal mucus as the fluid of the Lungs; the Lungs' association with the skin and outward manifestations in body hair; the Lungs and their special orifice, the nose

2.5.1 Relation to melancholy

The influence of melancholy and grief on the physiological activities of human body are similar, thus both of them are associated with the Lungs. Both melancholy or grief are considered emotional reactions that are not a positive stimulation and which may continuously consume Qi. Because the Lungs are in charge of Qi, it is easily impaired by melancholy. Equally, when Lung-Qi is deficient, the human body is susceptible to experiencing melancholy and grief because the body has a decreased ability to endure external stressors.

2.5.2 Nasal mucus as the fluid of the Lungs

Nasal mucus has the function of moistening the nostrils. Under normal condition, it should not flow out of the nose. When pathogenic Cold attacks the Lungs, a running nose results. When pathogenic Heat attacks the Lungs, yellow, thick and turbid discharge occurs. Lung Dryness is manifested as dryness of the nasal cavity.

2.5.3 The Lungs' association with the skin

Skin, sweat glands and body hair make up most of the body surface and depend on the warming, nourishing and moistening of defensive Qi and Body Fluid. Sweat glands are known as the 'valves of air'. These pores are not only the site for the excretion of sweat, but also for the exchange of air inside and outside the body, which is carried out by the Lungs' dispersing and descending functions.

2.5.4 The Lungs' special orifice is the nose

The nose and the larynx are the doors of respiration. The olfaction of the nose and the articulation of the larynx both depend on the action of Lung-Qi.

3. THE SPLEEN

In terms of Five Elements theory, the Spleen belongs to Earth, is the source of Qi and Blood transformation, and also the production of Qi and Blood, and is 'the organ in charge of the storehouse of food'. The Spleen has its specific orifice in the mouth and its outward manifestations in the lips. The Spleen is related to thinking, and saliva is the fluid of the Spleen. It dominates muscles and limbs. The Spleen is related externally and internally with the Stomach.

The main physiological functions of the Spleen are as follows.

3.1 Transportation and transformation

The Spleen functions physiologically in the transformation of food and Water into Essence, and in transportation of the essential substance to all parts of body, including the transformation and transportation of food and water.

Transportation and transformation of food: This refers to the digestion and absorption of food. The transformation of food into Essence is dependent on this function of the Spleen. *Plain Questions* states:

After food and drink enter the Stomach, they are digested and transformed into food Essence, and then transmitted upward to the Spleen, which disperses the Essence upward to the Lungs, and the Lungs regulate water pathways downward to the Bladder. And by doing so Body Fluid is finally disseminated to all parts of the body along all the meridians and collaterals.

It explains that the absorption of nutrient materials from food relies on the transportation and distribution of Essence by the Spleen, and this is the meaning of the statement in *Plain Questions*, 'the Spleen dominates the Body Fluid transmitted from the Stomach.'

Transportation and transformation of Water: The Spleen transports excess water in food Essence to the Lungs and Kidneys. Through Qi activities of the Lungs and Kidneys, the excess water is transformed into sweat and urine and discharged from the body. Therefore, Spleen dysfunction will result in water retention inside the body and lead to pathological productions such as Damp, Phlegm and fluid, even oedema. Hence, *Plain Questions* states: 'All Dampness with swelling and fullness is ascribed to the Spleen.' It means that Spleen deficiency gives rise to Damp, the Spleen is the source of Phlegm, and Spleen deficiency leads to oedema.

Transformation and transportation of food and Water is closely related to water metabolism. Transformation and transportation is the main physiological function of the Spleen, which plays a critical role in the entire vital activity of the human body. Hence, the Spleen and Stomach are regarded as 'the acquired foundation of life' and the source of producing Qi and Blood. Therefore, in terms of prevention and healthcare, attention should be paid not only to diet and nutrition, but also to protection of the Spleen and Stomach.

The process of food digestion and absorption is illustrated in Figure 2.6.

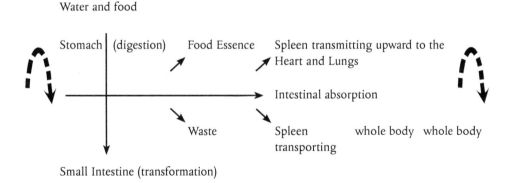

Figure 2.6: The process of food digestion and absorption

3.2 Spleen ascending clear Essence

'Clear' refers to the nutrient substances of water and food. Ascending clear Essence means the absorption, and upper distribution to the Heart, Lungs, head and eyes of the nutrient substances of water and food, whereupon substances can be transformed into Qi and Blood to nourish the whole body through the functions of the Heart and Lungs. So the Spleen is healthy when Spleen-Qi is ascending. The ascension of Spleen-Qi maintains the relatively fixed position of the internal organs, protecting them from prolapse. Dysfunction of Spleen-Qi in ascending due to Spleen-Qi deficiency leads to the failure to nourish the head and eyes, and to produce Qi and Blood Lassitude, dizziness, blurred vision, diarrhoea, etc can occur, there is 'prolapse of Qi in the Middle Burner' and in severe cases, such as prolonged diarrhoea or dysentery, prolapse of the internal organs including the rectum, stomach, kidneys and uterus, etc.

3.3 The Spleen controls the Blood

The Spleen has the function of keeping the Blood circulating inside the vessels and preventing it from extravasation. If Spleen-Qi becomes insufficient, the Qi cannot control the Blood, and Blood that flows outside the vessels will cause bleeding syndromes such as hemafecia, haematuria, functional uterus bleeding, etc., which can all occur as a result of the Spleen being unable to control Blood. In fact, the function of the Spleen to control Blood is through the controlling ability of Qi. And the Spleen is the foundation of Qi and Blood. When the function of the Spleen in transportation and transformation is good, Qi and Blood will be ample, the controlling ability of Qi will be strong, Blood will circulate inside the vessels, and bleeding will not occur; when the function of the Spleen in transportation and transformation is weak, the controlling ability of Qi will be not strong, so Qi will not control Blood and bleeding will occur.

3.4 The emotion of the Spleen is meditation; the fluid of the Spleen is saliva; the Spleen dominates the muscles and four limbs; the Spleen opens into the mouth and the outward manifestation of Spleen is in the lips

3.4.1 The emotion of the Spleen is meditation

Meditation or thinking is a type of emotion of the body. Meditation is the emotion of the Spleen, and combines with the function of the Heart to house the Mind. Normal meditation has no harmful effect on body physiology, but over-meditation can disturb the normal physiological activities of the body and cause difficulties in the flow of Qi and Qi stagnation.

3.4.2 The fluid of the Spleen is saliva

Saliva is the fluid of the mouth, and is the clear and dilute part of sputum. Its functions include protecting oral mucosa and moistening the oral cavity. Much saliva is secretes during food intake, so that it can promote the swallowing and digesting of food. Normally, saliva circulates upward to mouth but does not dribble out from the mouth. Disharmony of the Spleen and the Stomach can rapidly increase the amount of saliva so that saliva will come out of the mouth.

3.4.3 The Spleen dominates the muscles and four limbs

The Spleen and the Stomach are the foundation of Qi and Blood. The muscles of the whole body depend upon nourishment given by the functioning of the Spleen and Stomach in transportation and transformation of food and water; when this function is good, the muscles will be strong, otherwise they will be weak and atrophic. So there is a theory that 'Wei syndrome is treated only by points from the Yangming Meridian.'

3.4.4 The Spleen opens into the mouth

This means that appetite relates to the function of the Spleen in transportation and transformation. Normal appetite depends on normal Spleen-Qi in ascending and Stomach-Qi in descending. When the function of the Spleen in transportation and transformation is good, the appetite will be normal. Otherwise, abnormal appetite sensations such as a tasteless sweetish taste, a sticky mouth, or a bitter taste in the mouth will occur.

3.4.5 Outward manifestations of the Spleen are in the lips

The Spleen is the foundation of Qi and Blood. Red and moistened lips, or their absence, can reflect the status of Qi and Blood in the body and also respond to the functioning of the Spleen and Stomach in the transportation and transformation of food and water.

4. THE LIVER

The Liver belongs to Wood in terms of the Five Elements, and dominates moving and ascending. It is called the 'General Organ'.

The Liver opens into the eyes, and its outward manifestations are in the nails. The emotion of the Liver is anger, the fluid of the Liver is tears, and the Liver has an internal and external relationship with the Gallbladder.

The main physiological functions of the Liver are as follows.

4.1 The Liver maintains the free flowing of Qi

The Liver is responsible for the harmonious and unobstructed functional activities of the human body. When the function of the Liver in maintaining the free flowing of Qi is normal, Qi circulation will be good, Qi and Blood will be harmonized, and the activities of the Zang Fu organs and tissues will be normal and peaceful. If the function of the Liver in maintaining the free flowing of Qi is abnormal, the Liver-Qi will be obstructed, and depression, and sighing, etc. will occur; if the function of the Liver in maintaining free flowing Qi is excessively strong, the Liver-Qi will perversely run up to cause emotional hyperactivity manifested by irritability, easy anger, and insomnia with disturbed dreams.

This function manifests in the following ways.

Regulating Qi activity: Qi activity refers to ascending and descending, the coming and going of Qi. Body movement totally depends upon Qi activity. And as the Liver dominates ascending and moving, it is an important factor in the free flow of Qi. When the Liver fails to maintain the free flow of Qi, the ascending of Qi will be insufficient, and Qi will be obstructed; when the Liver forcefully ascends Qi, the descending of Qi will be insufficient, and the movement of Liver-Qi will be perversely upwards; if Blood follows the upward perversion of Qi, bleeding will occur; dysfunction of the Liver in maintaining the free flow of Qi can disturb Blood circulation and fluid metabolism, and pathological substances such as Blood stasis and Phlegm can occur.

Promoting digestion by the Spleen and Stomach: Harmony and balance of ascending clear function of the Spleen and the descending turbid function of the Stomach closely relates with the function of the Liver in maintaining the free flow of Qi. If the function of the Liver in maintaining the free flow of Qi is abnormal, the ascending clear function of the Spleen will be affected, and will be manifested in the upper part of the body as dizziness, and in the lower part of the body in diarrhoea. If the function of the Liver in maintaining the free flow of Qi is abnormal, the descending turbid function of the Stomach will be affected – in the upper part of the body this will be manifested in vomiting and belching, in the middle part in epigastric and abdominal distention and pain, and in the lower part of the body in constipation. The function of the Liver in maintaining the free flow of Qi also relates to the secretion and excretion of bile. Bile is formed by a part of the Qi in the Liver, and the secretion and excretion of bile manifests the function of the Liver in maintaining the free flow of Qi. When Liver-Qi stagnation affects the secretion and excretion of bile, then symptoms such as hypochondriac distention and pain, a bitter taste in the mouth, poor appetite and even jaundice, will occur.

The function of the Liver in maintaining the free flow of Qi can promote digestion by the Spleen and Stomach (see Figure 2.8).

Normal:

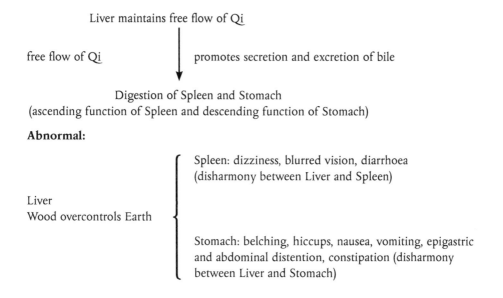

Liver maintains free flow of Qi

free flow of Qi ↓ promotes secretion and excretion of bile

Digestion of Spleen and Stomach
(ascending function of Spleen and descending function of Stomach)

Abnormal:

Liver
Wood overcontrols Earth {

Spleen: dizziness, blurred vision, diarrhoea
(disharmony between Liver and Spleen)

Stomach: belching, hiccups, nausea, vomiting, epigastric
and abdominal distention, constipation (disharmony
between Liver and Stomach)

Figure 2.8: The function of the Liver in the flow of Qi

Regulating emotional activity: Emotional activity is governed by the physiological function of the Heart in housing the Mind, but it also has a close relationship with the function of the Liver in maintaining the free flow of Qi. Normal emotional activity relies on normal circulation of Qi and Blood, and the Liver has the function of maintaining the free flow of Qi. So when the function of the Liver in maintaining the free flow of Qi is normal, Qi and Blood will be harmonized and emotional activity will be good; if the function of the Liver in maintaining the free flow of Qi is inadequate, Liver-Qi will stagnate and the emotion will be depressive; if the Liver forcefully ascends Qi, the emotion will manifest as easily irritable and angry.

Promoting male sperm, female ovulation and menstruation: All of the sperm, ovulation and menstruation functions relate to the function of the Liver in maintaining the free flow of Qi. If the function of the Liver in maintaining the free flow of Qi becomes abnormal, pathological phenomena such as spermatorrhoea and irregular menstruation, etc. will occur.

4.2 Liver storing Blood

The Liver has the function of storing Blood and regulating the volume of Blood in circulation in order to prevent bleeding; the fact that the Liver stores a certain volume of Blood can forcefully restrict the ascending of Liver Yang; retain the free flow of the Liver; and prevent bleeding. If the Liver does not store Blood, Liver Blood will not be sufficient, Liver-Qi will perversely rise, and bleeding syndromes such as haematemesis, heavy menses and functional uterus bleeding will occur.

Figure 2.9 illustrates the function of the Liver in storing Blood.

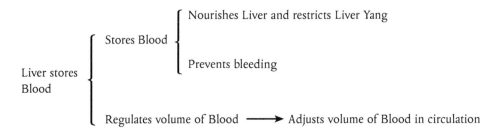

Figure 2.9: The function of the Liver in storing Blood

Liver adjusts the volume of Blood in circulation: Normally, the volume of Blood in every part of body is relatively balanced. But the volume of Blood circulating in various parts of the body changes according to greater or lesser physiological needs, emotions and climate. During vigorous movement and emotional excitement, Blood is released from the Liver to increase the volume of Blood in circulation for physiological needs; during rest and quietness, the volume of Blood required decreases, and part of the Blood remains in the Liver.

4.3 The emotion of the Liver is anger; the fluid of the Liver is tears; the Liver controls the tendons and the Liver opens into the eye

4.3.1 The emotion of Liver is anger

Anger is an emotional change due to excitement. In general, it is regarded as a bad stimulation. Anger can cause Qi and Blood perversely to attack upwards. Because the Liver has the function of maintaining the free flow of Qi, it controls the ascending and dispersing of Yang Qi, and the emotion of the Liver is anger. Severe anger causes Liver Yang Qi forcefully to ascend and disperses, and as a result Liver Yin Blood becomes deficient. When Liver Yang Qi forcefully attacks upwards, anger will easily occur after only slight stimulation.

4.3.2 The fluid of the Liver is tears

The Liver opens into the eye, and tears comes from the eye; tears have the function of moistening the eye and protecting the physiological functions of the eye. Normally, tears stay in the eye, but when a foreign object comes into the eye, the secretion of large amounts of tears can moisten the eye and wash out the foreign object. Pathologically, the secretion of tears can be abnormal producing watery eyes.

4.3.3 The Liver controls the tendons

By tendon we mean the tendon membrane that attaches to the bone and accumulates on the joints. It is a type of tissue that links with joints and muscles. The contraction and relaxation of tendon and muscle create the flexion, extension and rotation of limbs and joints. Ample Liver Blood can nourish the tendons, so movement is flexible and strong. Energy to create body movement comes from the function of the Liver in storing Blood and adjust in the volume of Blood in circulation. When Liver-Qi and Blood become deficient, the tendon membrane cannot be nourished, and there is a limitation on the joints in movement, so 'extreme fatigue and tiredness arises from the dysfunction of the Liver in storing the Blood'; if Liver Yin Blood is deficient, it cannot nourish tendons, and symptoms including trembling of hands and feet, numbness of the limbs, limitation of joints in flexion and extension, and even convulsion will occur, so 'various kinds of Wind leading to tremor and dizziness are related to dysfunction of the Liver'.

4.3.4 The Liver manifests in the nails

Both fingernails and toenails are the extension of the tendons. Ample or weak Liver Blood can affect the quality of the nails. When Liver Blood is sufficient, nails are strong, lustrous and rosy; when Liver Blood becomes deficient, nails become soft and thin, withered, or even deformed and chipped.

4.3.5 The Liver opens into the eye

The eye is also described in terms of brightness and is the visual organ. The Liver Meridian runs upwards to link with the eye system. Vision relies on the Liver to flow the Qi freely and to store Blood, so the Liver opens into the eye. Whether the Liver function is normal or not often reflects in the eye. When Liver Yin Blood is deficient, dryness of the eye, unclear vision and even night blindness can happen; Wind and Heat in the Liver meridian can cause redness, itching and pain in the eyes;

a flare-up of Liver Fire can lead to cornea conjunctivitis; and an attack upwards of Liver Yang can cause heterotropia and the eyeball to turn upwards abnormally.

5. THE KIDNEYS

The Kidneys belong to Water in terms of the Five Elements. The Kidneys store 'congenital Essence' and are the root of Yin and Yang in the Zang Fu organs (the source of life) so they are called 'the organ for construction'. The Kidneys open into the ear, dominating anterior and posterior orifices, and manifest in the hair. The emotion of the Kidneys is the state of being frightened, and fear. The fluid of the Kidneys is saliva and the Kidneys have an interior and exterior relationship to the Bladder.

The main physiological functions of the Kidneys are as follows.

5.1 Kidneys store Essence and dominate growth, development and reproduction

Kidneys store Essence: The Kidneys can store Essence so that Essence will not be lost and affect the growth, development and reproduction of the body. Essence is the basic material of the human body and of many of its functional activities. Kidney Essence consists of two parts: congenital and acquired. Congenital Essence is inherited from the parents. Acquired Essence is transformed from the essential substances of food and Water by the Spleen and Stomach, and is the remaining part of Essence produced by Zang Fu physiological activities after metabolism. Although the source of congenital Essence and acquired Essence is different, congenital and acquired Essence are both stored in the Kidneys; the two essences rely on and promote each other. Before birth, congenital Essence has prepared the material base for acquired Essence. After birth, acquired Essence constantly replenishes congenital Essence. Congenital Essence and acquired Essence integrate into Kidney Essence in the Kidney to dominate growth, development and reproduction, as shown in Figure 2.10.

Kidney Yin and Kidney Yang: Kidney Essence includes Kidney Yin and Kidney Yang. Kidney Yin has the function of nourishing and moistening the body; Kidney Yang has the function of warming up the body. Kidney Yin and Kidney Yang are the root of Yin–Yang in every organ; together they maintain the relative balance of Yin–Yang in every organ. When this relative balance is disturbed, Kidney Yin deficiency with symptoms of fever, dizziness, tinnitus, weakness and soreness of the low back and knee joints, spermatorrhoea, will occur and the body of the tongue will be red with scanty coating, or Kidney Yang deficiency with symptoms of lassitude, chills, cold sensation of the four limbs, cold pain and weakness of the low back and knee joints, clear and profuse urination or enuresis and incontinence of urination, the body of the tongue will be pale, sexual dysfunction, and oedema, etc. will occur. An imbalance of Kidney Yin–Yang can cause Yin–Yang imbalance in other organs, such as when Kidney Yin fails to nourish the Lungs, then there is both Lung and Kidney Yin deficiency with symptoms of sore throat, dry cough, tidal fever and feverish sensations; when the Kidneys fail to warm up the Spleen, then there is both Heart and Kidney Yang deficiency with symptoms of diarrhoea at day break, diarrhoea, etc; and Heart and Kidney Yang deficiency with symptoms of palpitation, sweating and shortness of breathing, etc. On the other hand, an imbalance of Yin–Yang in other organs can cause an imbalance of Yin–Yang in the Kidneys, as 'prolonged diseases disturb the Kidneys'. So both Kidney Yin and Kidney Yang rely on Kidney Essence as their material base. In fact, Kidney Yin deficiency and Kidney Yang deficiency are due to Kidney Essence deficiency. When Kidney Yin reaches a certain level of deficiency, Kidney Yang will be affected and both Yin and Yang in the Kidneys will be deficient; it is 'Yin injury disturbing Yang'; when Kidney Yang reaches a certain level of deficiency, Kidney Yin will be affected and both Yin and Yang in the Kidneys will be deficient: this is 'Yang injury disturbing Yin'.

Kidney-Qi deficiency: Under certain conditions, although Kidney Essence is deficient, the imbalance of Yin–Yang is not obvious, and so it is also named Kidney Essence deficiency.

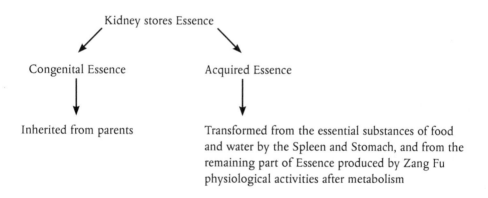

Figure 2.10: Congenital Essence and acquired Essence integrate into Kidney Essence

5.2 The Kidneys dominate water metabolism

The Qi activity of the Kidneys play an extremely important role in regulating the distribution and metabolism of Body Fluid. Normally, water is first received by the Stomach, and then transmitted by the Spleen to the Lungs, which disperse it and cause it to descend. The evaporation and Qi activity of Kidney Essence dominate all metabolic processes. The functions of the Lungs and Spleen on Body Fluid rely on the evaporation and Qi activity of Kidney Essence; the formation and excretion of urine plays an important role in maintaining the balance of Body Fluid metabolism, which directly relates to the Kidneys, so the Kidneys dominate water metabolism. If the Qi activity of the Kidneys is abnormal, 'opening and closing' of the Kidneys will be also abnormal, pathological symptoms of disturbance of urine such as scanty urination and oedema will occur and then abnormal Qi activity cannot dominate water metabolism, so pathological symptoms including profuse and clear urination, and large amounts of urination will occur.

The process of fluid metabolism is shown in Figure 2.11.

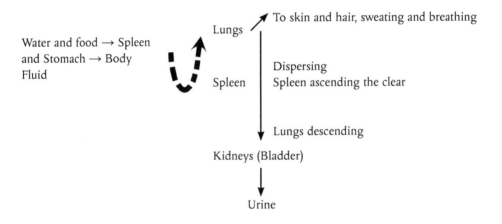

Figure 2.11: The process of fluid metabolism

5.3 The Kidneys receive Qi

The Kidneys receive clear Qi inhaled by the Lungs to prevent shallow breathing and maintain the normal Qi exchange throughout the internal and external parts of the body. Clear Qi inhaled by the Lungs can maintain a certain depth when the Kidneys receive Qi. The function of the Kidneys in receiving Qi is a phenomenon of the storing function of the Kidneys manifested in respiration.

Dysfunction of the Kidneys in receiving Qi: If Kidney Essence is deficient, so that the Kidneys cannot receive Qi and thus help the Lungs maintain depth of respiration, then shallow breathing, more exhaling than inhaling, or shortness of breathing after movement, etc. can occur.

5.4 The emotion of the Kidneys is fear; the fluid of the Kidneys is saliva; the Kidneys dominate bone, manufacture marrow and manifest in the hair; the Kidneys open into the ear and dominate the anterior and posterior orifices

5.4.1 The emotion of the Kidneys is fear

Fear is a mental condition in which a person is afraid of something. Fear is similar to being frightened. Being frightened arises unconsciously because it is caused by something sudden or unexpected. Fear is an emotion related to knowing what will happen but being afraid of it. 'Fear causes Qi to descend' means that Qi is compelled downward because the Qi activity in the Upper Burner is obstructed by fear, when the person is fearful. This causes distention in the Lower Burner, enuresis; 'fright causes a confusion of Qi' means that there is irritability, but no idea what to do because of the sudden onset.

5.4.2 The fluid of the Kidney is saliva

Saliva is fluid of the mouth, the sticky part of sputum. Saliva is transformed by Kidney Essence and swallowed but not spat out; it has the function of nourishing Kidney Essence. A large amount of saliva or prolonged saliva production can easily consume Kidney Essence. As the ancient physicians said, when the tongue touches the palate, then saliva is swallowed when the mouth is full.

5.4.3 The Kidneys dominate bone, manufacture marrow to fill up the brain and manifest in the hair

The function of the Kidneys to dominate bone and manufacture marrow is an important component part of the Kidney Essence that dominates the development and reproduction of the body. The marrow nourishes the growth and development of bone. The late-closing fontanelle of the infant, the soft and weak bones of infants, the bone fragility of older people and the ease with which their bones fracture, all relate to Kidney Essence deficiency leading to empty bone and marrow. Marrow consists of bone marrow, spinal marrow and brain marrow, all of which are transformed by Kidney Essence. The changing strengths and weaknesses of Kidney Essence can affect the growth and development of bone, and the sufficiency and development of spinal marrow and brain marrow. The spinal marrow ascends to connect with the brain, which is formed by the accumulation of marrow, so the brain is 'the Sea of Marrow'. When Kidney Essence is sufficient, the Sea of Marrow can be nourished and the development of the brain is healthy; if Kidney Essence is deficient, it cannot nourish the Sea of Marrow, and then pathological change relating to insufficiency of the Sea of Marrow can occur.

Growth or loss of hair, and the lustre or withering of hair occurred as a result of the nourishment given by Kidney Essence and Blood, 'the hair is the tip of the Blood'. Throughout the prime of life, the Kidney Essence Blood is sufficient, so the hair is lustrous; in old age, the Kidney Essence Blood becomes deficient, and the hair turns white and falls out: this is normal. But clinically, dry and falling hair that terms white at a young age indicates Kidney Essence deficiency and Blood deficiency.

5.4.4 The Kidneys open into the ear and dominate the anterior and posterior orifices

The ear is the hearing organ. The function of the ear in dominating hearing relies on nourishment by the Kidney Essence. When the Kidney Essence is sufficient, the Sea of Marrow (the brain) can be nourished, hearing is acute and decision-making power is strong; otherwise, Kidney Essence deficiency fails to nourish the Sea of Marrow, hearing ability is decreased or tinnitus, even deafness, can result.

The anterior orifice refers to the urethra and genitalia, the posterior orifice refers to the anus. The anterior orifice is the organ of urination and reproduction, the posterior orifice is the passage for excreting faeces. Although the discharge of urine is a function of the Bladder, it also relies on the Qi activity of the Kidneys. Dysfunction of the Qi activity of the Kidneys can result in frequent urination, urgent urination, enuresis, incontinence of urination, scanty urination or anuria; the Kidneys also dominate reproduction. Excretion of faeces occurs through the function of Large Intestine in transforming and transporting waste material, which also relates to the Qi activity of the Kidneys. If Kidney Yin becomes deficient, the intestinal fluid is dry, which can result in constipation; if Kidney Yang is deficient, dysfunction of the Qi activity of the Kidneys can cause constipation or diarrhoea, depending on the type of Yang deficiency; dysfunction of the Kidneys in storing can result in prolonged diarrhoea and prolapse of the rectum.

III. THE SIX FU ORGANS

The main physiological functions of the six Fu organs are described below.

The six Fu organs: The general term for the Gallbladder, Stomach, Small Intestine, Large Intestine, Bladder, and the Triple Burner.

Seven gates: There are seven gates that food and water pass through from intake to excretion, and these seven gates have individual functions in accomplishing digestion and the absorption of food and water. *Classic on Medical Problems* said:

lip is the flying gate, teeth are the house gate, epiglottis is the respiratory gate, Stomach is the cardia, lower outlet of Stomach is the pylorus, Large Intestine and Small Intestine are ileocaecal conjunction, anus is the gate to excrete waste material.

Seven gates for digestion and absorption of food and water

	Name	Function
Lips	Flying gate	Take in food and water
Teeth	House gate	Chew food so that it can be swallowed
Epiglottis	Respiratory gate	Separate swallowed food for the Stomach from air for Lungs
Stomach	Cardia	Receives food into the Stomach
Stomach/Small Intestine	Pylorus	Allows processed food to move from the Stomach to the Small Intestines
Small Intestine/Large Intestine	Ileocaecal conjunction	The gate between the Small and Large Intestine
Anus	Excreting	The gate through which the solid waste products of food leave the body

The lips of the mouth can freely open and close, so this is the flying gate. Food can be swallowed after chewing by the teeth, so the teeth are the house gate. The epiglottis is the place of connection between the oesophagus and the trachea and is the necessary entrance through which food descends to the oesophagus; it is also the gate to inhale and exhale, so it is the respiratory gate. The cardia is the upper outlet of the Stomach; the Stomach is the place where food is received; the connection between the lower outlet of the Stomach and the upper outlet of Small Intestine is the pylorus; the connection between the lower outlet of the Small Intestine and the upper outlet of the Large Intestine is the ileocaecal conjunction; the anus is the gate to excreting wasted material. When the functions of any one of the seven gates becomes abnormal, the functions of ingesting, digesting, absorbing and excreting food will be affected.

1. THE GALLBLADDER

The Gallbladder is the head of the six Fu organs, the organ in charge of making decisions, and is also one of the Extraordinary Fu organs. The Gallbladder has both an internal and external relationship with the Liver. Its main function is to store and excrete bile. Bile can help the digestion of food, so the Gallbladder is therefore one of the six Fu organs. But, since the Gallbladder does not receive Water or food, and does store bile, it is unlike the other Fu organs, and for this reason it is also classified as one of the 'extra Fu organs'.

2. THE STOMACH

The Stomach is located in the epigastrium. It is divided into three parts: the upper part, the middle part and the lower part. It is also known as the 'store of food and water', or 'the sea of food and water'.

Its main function is to receive and break down food and water; and to transmit these downwards. The Stomach is in harmony when the Qi of the Stomach descends.

2.1 The Stomach receives and breaks down food and water

The Stomach receives and contains food and Water, then initially digest it in order to break it down. Food passes through the oesophagus and is received by the Stomach and thus the Stomach is 'the store of food and water', or 'the sea of food and water'. The physiological functions of the body and the transformation of Qi and Blood rely on nourishment given by food and water, so the Stomach is also described as the 'sea of Qi and Blood, food and water'. The Stomach contains and breaks down food and water, and then transmits these down to the Small Intestine. Its essential substances are then transported and transformed by the Spleen to supply the whole body. So the function of the Stomach in receiving and containing food and water combines with the function of Spleen in transporting and transforming food and water into essential substances and Qi, Blood, and Body Fluids that nourish the whole body.

2.2 The Stomach transmits downwards and is in harmony when the Qi of the Stomach descends

The Stomach transmits decomposed food down to the Small Intestine for further digestion and absorption. The transmitting-down function of the Stomach also includes the Small Intestine transmiting the residue of food down to the Large Intestine where the Large Intestine forms the remainder into faeces to be excreted. That the turbid element of the processed food should descend is essential to the whole process of receiving and containing food.

If the descending function is disturbed, turbid Qi goes up, the symptoms of which include a foul smell in the mouth, epigastric distention or pain, and constipation;

moveover, if the descending function is disturbed, Stomach-Qi can perversely attack upwards, causing symptoms such as belching, acid regurgitation, nausea, vomiting, and hiccups.

3. THE SMALL INTESTINE

The main functions of the Small Intestine are reception, digestion, and separation of clear from turbid.

3.1 Reception and digestion

The Small intestine receives the food that is initially digested by the Stomach. This food then stays some time in the Small Intestine for further digestion.

3.2 Separation of clear from turbid

This involves the following:

- The separation of the essential substances of food and water from the residue of the food after digestion in the Small Intestine.

- Absorption of the essential substance of food, and transmitting the residue of the food to the Large Intestine.

- The Small Intestine in absorbing large amounts of water as it absorbs food, described as the 'Small Intestine dominating fluid'. The function of the Small Intestine in separating clear from turbid also relates to the amount of urine. If there is a dysfunction of the Small Intestine in separating clear from turbid, symptoms such as watery stools and scanty urination can occur. Clinically, there is a treatment principle involving 'promotion of the function of the Small Intestine in separating clear from turbid to benefit faeces'.

4. THE LARGE INTESTINE

The main function of the Large Intestine is transportation and transformation of waste material. The Large Intestine receives the waste material sent down from the Small Intestine, absorbs its fluid content, and forms the remainder into faeces to be excreted through the anus.

The function of the Large Intestine in transportation is an extension of the function of Stomach in descending the turbid, and also relates to the function of the Lungs in descending and dispersing. Furthermore, the function of the Large

Intestine in transportation relates to the Qi activity of the Kidneys, so 'Kidneys dominate anterior and posterior orifices'.

5. THE BLADDER

The main function of the Bladder is to store and excrete urine.

Urine is transformed by Body Fluid, formed through the Qi activity of the Kidneys and descends to the Bladder. Urine is discharged from the body when a sufficient quantity has been accumulated, and so the Bladder is called the 'Water organ'.

The function of the Bladder in storing and excreting urine totally relies on the Qi activity of the Kidneys. In fact, the Qi activity of the Bladder belongs to the evaporation and Qi activity of the Kidneys. Diseases of the Bladder manifest in frequent urination, urgent urination, painful urination; or difficult urination, dribbling urination, even anuria; or enuresis, and even incontinence of urination.

6. THE TRIPLE BURNER

The Triple Burner is divided into three parts: the Upper, Middle and Lower Burners.

The Triple Burner does not have a definite physical position in the body in the same way as the other organs: it has a name but is invisible. It is a big Fu organ distributed across the cavity of the chest and abdomen. Its main functions are:

To govern various forms of Qi and serve Qi activity: The Triple Burner is the pathway for ascending and descending Qi, and for the movement of Qi in and out of the cavities; it is the place of Qi activity. Primary Qi is the most fundamental Qi of the body and the root of primary Qi is in the Kidneys. Primary Qi is distributed to the whole body through the Triple Burner – as *Classic on Medical Problems* says, 'the Triple Burner is the ambassador of primary Qi'.

The passage of water metabolism: The Triple Burner regulates the passage of water and the system of water circulation, so it is the passage of water ascending and descending, entering and leaving the cavities of the body. The water metabolism of the whole body is performed by organs such as the Lungs, Spleen and Stomach, Intestines, Kidneys, Bladder, etc. working in coordination. The Triple Burner controls the passages where this is performed, including the ascending and descending functions and the movement in and out of the cavities. If the Triple Burner cannot regulate the passage of water, the function of the Lungs, Spleen and Kidneys in distributing water and regulating the water metabolism cannot be performed. So coordinating, and balancing water metabolism is described as the 'Qi activity of the Triple Burner'.

IV. THE EXTRAORDINARY FU ORGANS

The extra Fu organs comprise the brain, marrow, bones, vessels, Gallbladder and uterus. The empty nature of their forms is similar to the forms of the Fu organs but their functions in storing Essence and Qi are similar to the physiological functions of the Zang organs. Apart from the Gallbladder, the other Extraordinary Fu organs do not have an internal–external relationship with other organs or properties of the Five Elements.

1. THE BRAIN

The Brain is formed by a collection of marrow, so the 'brain is the Sea of Marrow', and 'the head is the residence of intelligence'. The brain is related to the activity of thinking.

2. THE UTERUS

The uterus presides over menstruation and nourishes the foetus. The uterus is the organ responsible for the onset of menstruation, for pregnancy and for the birth of the foetus, all of which are complicated processes. These processes have a close relationship with Tian Gui (see below), the Thoroughfare and Conception Vessels, and the Zang organs Heart, Liver, and Spleen.

2.1 The Functions of Tian Gui

Tian Gui: This substance appear when essential Qi accumulates to a certain amount, and its the physiological function is to promote gonadal development to maturity. With the promotion of Tian Gui, the female genital organs can develop and mature, menstruation can occur in preparation for pregnancy and the birth of the foetus. Because Kidney Essence in older people decreases, Tian Gui also becomes deficient (even exhausted), and so menstruation and the possibility of giving birth cease.

2.2 Functions of the Thoroughfare and Conception Vessels

Both of these vessels originate from the uterus: the Thoroughfare Vessel runs parallel to the Kidney Meridian, links with the Yangming Meridian and functions to regulate the Qi and Blood of all the twelve regular meridians, so it is described at the 'Sea of Blood'; the Conception Vessel dominates the uterus, meets with the three Yin meridians of the foot on the lower abdomen and regulates the Qi of all the Yin meridians, so it is called the 'Sea of Yin Meridians'. When the Qi and Blood in the twelve regular meridians are ample, Qi and Blood can be infused into the uterus through the regulation of the Thoroughfare and Conception Vessels, and then menstruation can take place. The rise and fall of the Thoroughfare and Conception Vessels depends on the adjustment of Tian Gui. Clinically, dysfunction of the Thoroughfare and Conception Vessels can lead to irregular menstruation, infertility, etc.

2.3 Functions of the Heart, Liver, Spleen

The Heart dominates Blood and vessels, the Liver stores Blood, and the Spleen is concerned with the formation of Qi and Blood and controls the Blood. These three organs can regulate the formation and circulation of Blood. The coming of menstruation, pregnancy and the birth of a foetus all relate to nourishment through ample Qi and Blood, and the normal regulation of Blood, so menstruation has a relationship with the Heart, Liver and Spleen. Dysfunctions of the Liver in storing Blood, and the Spleen is controlling Blood can lead to heavy menses, a shortened cycle of menstruation, a prolonged menstrual period, even functional uterus bleeding; a dysfunction of the Spleen in producing Qi and Blood can cause menstrual Blood to be insufficient, so that very light menses, a prolonged cycle of menstruation, or amenorrhea can occur; when emotional changes disturb the function of the Heart in housing the Mind, or the Liver in allowing free flow of Qi, there is irregular menstruation.

V. THE RELATIONSHIPS AMONG THE ZANG AND FU ORGANS

1. THE RELATIONSHIP BETWEEN THE ZANG ORGANS

In ancient times, physicians mostly explained the relationships between the Zang organs in terms of interpromoting, interacting, overacting and counteracting. As a result of the continuously plentiful experiences of clinical practice, and the improvement in and development of theoretical systems, understanding the relationships between the Zang organs has gone beyond the range of mechanical circulation and interpromoting, interacting, overacting and counteracting of the Five Elements; it now mainly describes the coordination of body functional activities between the Zang organs – namely physical mutual coordination, and pathological mutual influence.

1.1 The Heart and Lungs

Both the Heart and the Lungs are situated in the Upper Burner, the Heart dominating Blood and the Lungs dominating Qi, so 'all of the Blood belong to the Heart' and 'all of the Qi belongs to the Lungs'. The relationship between the Heart and Lungs mainly manifests in mutual dependence and the mutual effect of Qi and Blood. The Lungs 'face to a hundred vessels' and has the function of descending and dispersing Qi. Blood will circulate when Qi circulates, so the function of the Lungs can help the Heart to circulate Blood. This is a necessary factor in keeping the Blood circulating normally, so 'Qi is the general of Blood'. In contrast, when the function of the Heart in dominating Blood is normal, Blood circulation will be good, Lung-Qi will be freely descended and dispersed, and the function of the Lungs in controlling respiration will be normal, so that 'exhalation relates to Heart and the Lungs'.

The physical and pathological relations of the Heart and the Lungs are described in Figure 2.11.

Physiology:

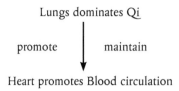

Lungs dominates Qi

promote   maintain

Heart promotes Blood circulation

Pathology:

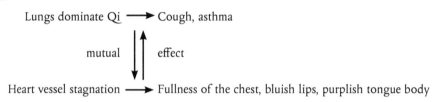

Lungs dominate Qi ⟶ Cough, asthma

mutual   effect

Heart vessel stagnation ⟶ Fullness of the chest, bluish lips, purplish tongue body

Figure 2.11: The physical and pathological relations of the Heart and the Lungs

1.2 The Heart and the Spleen

The Heart dominates Blood and the Spleen controls Blood; the Spleen is the foundation of Qi and Blood, and the relationship between the Heart and the Spleen manifests in the production and transportation of Blood.

The physical and pathological relations of the Heart and the Spleen are described in Figure 2.12.

Physiology:

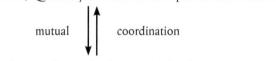

Heart dominates Blood, Qi activity of Heart involves production of Blood

mutual   coordination

Spleen produces Blood, controls Blood

Pathology:

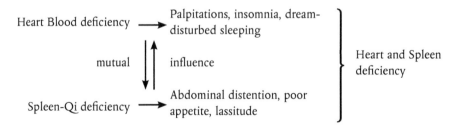

Heart Blood deficiency ⟶ Palpitations, insomnia, dream-disturbed sleeping

mutual   influence   } Heart and Spleen deficiency

Spleen-Qi deficiency ⟶ Abdominal distention, poor appetite, lassitude

Figure 2.12: The physical and pathological relations of the Heart and the Spleen

1.3 The Heart and the Liver

The Heart dominates Blood and the Liver stores Blood; the relationship between the Heart and the Liver manifests in Blood circulation and emotional activities.

The physical and pathological relations of the Heart and the Liver are described in Figure 2.13.

Physiology:

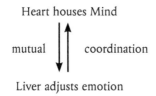

Heart dominates Blood

mutual   coordination

Liver stores Blood

Pathology:

Heart houses Mind

mutual   coordination

Liver adjusts emotion

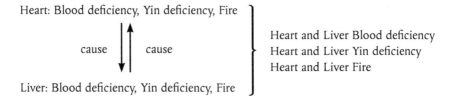

Heart: Blood deficiency, Yin deficiency, Fire ⎤
                   Heart and Liver Blood deficiency
cause   cause   Heart and Liver Yin deficiency
                   Heart and Liver Fire
Liver: Blood deficiency, Yin deficiency, Fire ⎦

Figure 2.13: The physical and pathological relations of the Heart and the Liver

1.4 The Heart and the Kidneys

In terms of the Five Elements, the Heart belongs to Fire; it is located in the upper part of the Triple Burner and is a Yang organ; in terms of the Five Elements the Kidneys belong to Water, they are located in the lower part of the Triple Burner and are a Yin organ. The relationship between the Heart and the Kidneys mainly manifests in balanced coordination, mutual dependence and control of movement up and down, Yin–Yang, Water and Fire.

The physical and pathological relations of the Heart and the Kidneys are described in Figure 2.14.

Physiology:

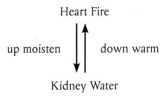

Pathology:

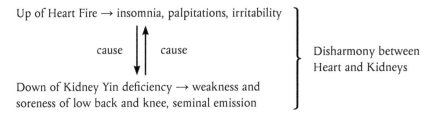

Figure 2.14: The physical and pathological relations of the Heart and the Kidneys

1.5 The Lungs and Spleen

The relationship between the Lungs and the Spleen manifests in the production of Qi and distribution of Body Fluid.

The physical and pathological relations of the Lung and the Spleen are described in Figure 2.15.

1.6 The Lungs and the Liver

The relationship between the Lungs and the Liver mainly manifests in regulation of Qi activities.

The physical and pathological relations of the Lungs and the Liver are described in Figure 2.16.

Physiology:

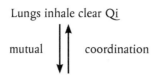

Lungs inhale clear Qi

mutual   coordination

Spleen transports and transforms food and water

Lung regulate water passage

mutual   coordination

Spleen transports and transforms water

Pathology:

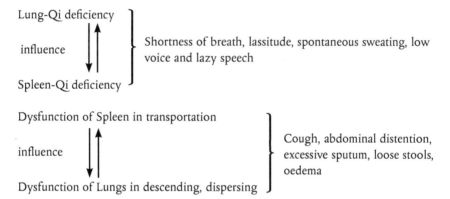

Lung-Qi deficiency

influence   } Shortness of breath, lassitude, spontaneous sweating, low voice and lazy speech

Spleen-Qi deficiency

Dysfunction of Spleen in transportation

influence   } Cough, abdominal distention, excessive sputum, loose stools, oedema

Dysfunction of Lungs in descending, dispersing

Figure 2.15: The physical and pathological relations of the Lungs and the Spleen

Physiology:

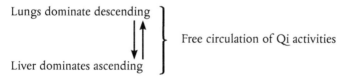

Lungs dominate descending

} Free circulation of Qi activities

Liver dominates ascending

Pathology:

Excessive Liver ascending, insufficient Lungs descending → Cough or even haemoptysis caused by upper perversion of Qi

Dysfunction of Lungs in descending, dysfunction of Liver in free flowing → Dull pain in chest and hypochondriac region, cough

Figure 2.16: The physical and pathological relations of the Lungs and the Liver

1.7 The Lungs and the Kidneys

The relationship between the Lungs and the Kidneys is mainly reflected in water metabolism and respiration.

The physiological and pathological relations of the Lungs and the Kidneys are described in Figure 2.17.

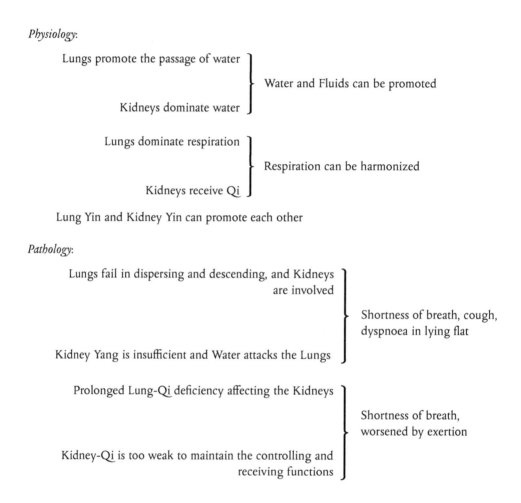

Physiology:

Lungs promote the passage of water
Kidneys dominate water
} Water and Fluids can be promoted

Lungs dominate respiration
Kidneys receive Qi
} Respiration can be harmonized

Lung Yin and Kidney Yin can promote each other

Pathology:

Lungs fail in dispersing and descending, and Kidneys are involved
Kidney Yang is insufficient and Water attacks the Lungs
} Shortness of breath, cough, dyspnoea in lying flat

Prolonged Lung-Qi deficiency affecting the Kidneys
Kidney-Qi is too weak to maintain the controlling and receiving functions
} Shortness of breath, worsened by exertion

Figure 2.17: The physical and pathological relations of the Lungs and the Kidneys

1.8 The Liver and the Spleen

The relationship between the Liver and the Spleen is mainly manifested in the transportation and transformation of water, and the storing and circulation of the Blood.

The physical and pathological relations of the Liver and the Spleen are described in Figure 2.18.

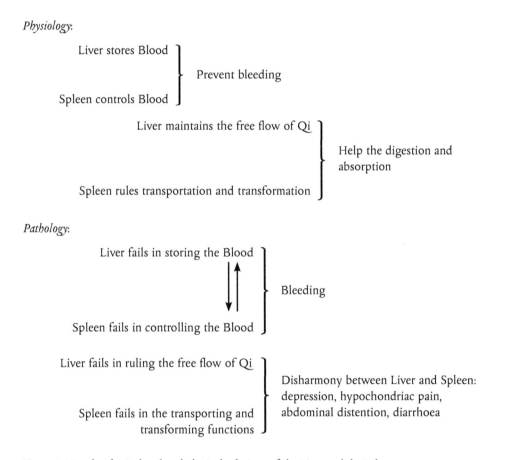

Physiology:

Liver stores Blood
Spleen controls Blood } Prevent bleeding

Liver maintains the free flow of Qi
Spleen rules transportation and transformation } Help the digestion and absorption

Pathology:

Liver fails in storing the Blood
Spleen fails in controlling the Blood } Bleeding

Liver fails in ruling the free flow of Qi
Spleen fails in the transporting and transforming functions } Disharmony between Liver and Spleen: depression, hypochondriac pain, abdominal distention, diarrhoea

Figure 2.18: The physical and pathological relations of the Liver and the Spleen

1.9 The Liver and the Kidneys

The relationship between the Liver and the Kidneys is, first, reflected in the interpromoting and intertransforming of the Essence and the Blood; second, the inter-inhibiting and interassisting relationship of the Liver ruling the free flow of Qi while the Kidneys dominates the storing function.

The physical and pathological relationship of the Liver and the Kidneys are shown in Figure 2.19.

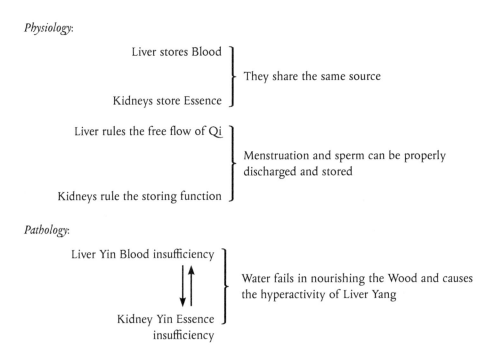

Physiology:

Liver stores Blood
Kidneys store Essence — They share the same source

Liver rules the free flow of Qi
Kidneys rule the storing function — Menstruation and sperm can be properly discharged and stored

Pathology:

Liver Yin Blood insufficiency
Kidney Yin Essence insufficiency — Water fails in nourishing the Wood and causes the hyperactivity of Liver Yang

Liver overrules the free flow of Qi → Storing function of the Kidneys is weak → Profuse menstruation for females, seminal emission and prospermia for males

Liver fails to rule the free flow of Qi → Storing function of the Kidneys is hyperactive → Amenorrhea for females and persistent erection without ejaculation for males

Figure 2.19: The physical and pathological relations of the Liver and the Kidneys

1.10 The Spleen and the Kidneys

The relationship between the Spleen and the Kidneys is mainly reflected in the interpromoting and interassisting between congenital and acquired conditions.

The physiological and pathological relations are described in Figure 2.20.

Physiology:

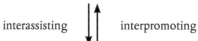

Spleen is the acquired foundation and rules the transportation
and transformation of water and fluids

interassisting   interpromoting

Kidneys are the congenital foundation and dominate water and fluids

Pathology:

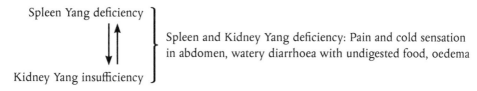

Spleen Yang deficiency

Kidney Yang insufficiency

Spleen and Kidney Yang deficiency: Pain and cold sensation
in abdomen, watery diarrhoea with undigested food, oedema

Figure 2.20: The physical and pathological relations of the Spleen and the Kidneys

2. THE RELATIONSHIP BETWEEN THE FU ORGANS

This is mainly reflected in their close relationship and cooperation in the process of the digestion, absorption and excretion of food and water.

Physiological: When food enters the Stomach, it is digested and sent down to the Small Intestine for further digestion – to separate the clear from the turbid. The clear part is the nutrient substance that can be sent to nourish the whole body by the Spleen. The turbid fluid part seeps into the Bladder and is excreted as urine by the evaporation function of Qi. The waste part of food is sent down to the Large Intestine and eliminated as faeces out of the body through its transportation and transformation function. This process of digestion, absorption and excretion also relies on the secretion of bile from the Gallbladder to help the digestion. The Triple Burner is the passage for the Body Fluids, and it can distribute the Body Fluids all over the body. The unified functions of the six Fu organs make them continuously receive, digest, transmit and excrete the water and food. The six Fu organs alternate from emptiness to fullness because they work well when they are not blocked. The six Fu organs should always be kept opened and clear instead of blocked.

Pathological: If excessive Heat in the Stomach consumes Body Fluids, then the function of the Large Intestine will be affected and constipation will result. Constipation may also affect the descending function of the Stomach, and then the reverse flow of Stomach-Qi may lead to symptoms such as nausea and vomiting.

3. THE RELATIONSHIP AMONG ZANG FU ORGANS

The relations of these organs are the relations between Yin–Yang, exterior and interior. The Zang organs pertain to Yin while the Fu organs pertain to Yang; they also relate to each other via the meridians.

3.1 The Heart and the Small Intestine

The Heart Meridian pertains to the Heart and connects to the Small Intestine Meridian; the Small Intestine Meridian pertains to the Small Intestine and connects to the Heart Meridian.

Pathologically, excessive Fire of the Heart Meridian may transmit pathogenic Heat to the Small Intestine, resulting in scanty urine, deep yellow urine, or pain and a burning sensation during urination; the Heat in the Small Intestine may ascend along the Meridian to affect the Heart, leading to symptoms such as mental restlessness, redness and ulceration of the tongue, etc.

3.2 The Lungs and the Large Intestine

The Lung and Large Intestine Meridians are related internally and externally. The descending function of the Lungs can help the Large Intestine to maintain its normal function of transmission; the normal transmission function of the Large Intestine also helps the Lungs carry out their normal function in descending.

Pathologically, excessive Heat in the Large Intestine can lead to the obstruction of the Fu organs' Qi, and affect the descending function of the Lungs, resulting in symptoms such as asthma, cough and fullness in the chest. If the Lungs fail to send down Body Fluids due to a dysfunction in descending, this can lead to symptoms such as difficult bowel movements, constipation or loose stools.

3.3 The Spleen and the Stomach

The Spleen and Stomach Meridians are related internally and externally. The Spleen transports and transforms the Body Fluids for the Stomach, and they work together to digest and absorb food and Water, and then send the nutrient substances all over the body.

Pathologically, they affect each other. Dysfunction of the Spleen in transportation and transformation can produce pathogenic dampness, and then the clear Qi cannot be ascended, so the receiving and descending functions of the Stomach will be affected, and symptoms such as poor appetite, vomiting, nausea, abdominal distention may appear. If there is improper food intake, or food retention in the Stomach, the Stomach loses its descending and harmonizing functions, which may affect the function of the Spleen in ascending the clear Qi, and transporting and transforming food and Water, and then symptoms such as abdominal distention and diarrhoea may occur.

3.4 The Liver and the Gallbladder

The Liver and Gallbladder Meridians are related internally and externally. Bile derives from the residue of the Liver-Qi, and the normal secretion function of the bile depends on the normal function of the Liver in freeing the flow of Qi. Liver dominates the idea, and Gallbladder dominates the decision – after getting an idea, the decision should be made. Therefore the Liver and Gallbladder have a very close relationship.

3.5 The Kidneys and the Bladder

The Kidneys and Bladder Meridians are related internally and externally. The functions of the Bladder in storing and discharging urine depend on the evaporation function of the Kidneys. When the Kidney-Qi is sufficient and the function normal, the Bladder opens and closes regularly, and then the water metabolism will be normal.

Pathologically, deficiency of Kidney-Qi, dysfunction of evaporation, or dysfunction of consolidation can result in incontinence, dysuria, enuresis or frequent urination.

CHAPTER 3

QI, BLOOD AND
BODY FLUIDS

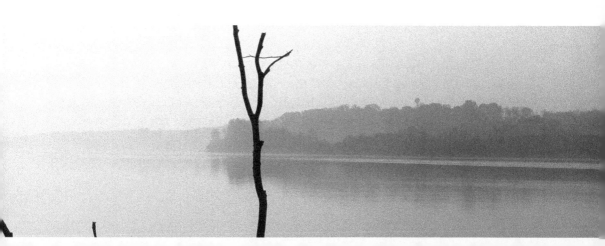

I. QI

Qi, Blood and Body Fluids are the fundamental substances of the human body. They are the material foundation for the physiological functions of the Zang Fu organs, tissues and meridians.

1. THE CONCEPT OF QI

Qi is the most basic substance of the human body, as well as the fundamental substance in maintaining the vital activities of the human body.

2. THE FORMATION OF QI

The Qi of the human body is derived from the congenital Essence of the parents, the nutrients of food (the Essence of food and water), and the clear Qi from the natural air. It is formed through the general physiological functions of organs such as the Lungs, Spleen and Kidneys, as shown in Figure 3.1.

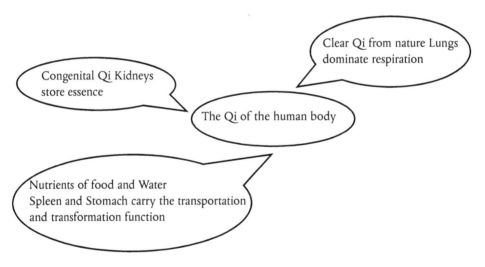

Figure 3.1: The formation of Qi

Qi is sufficient only when the physiological functions of the Kidneys, Spleen, Stomach and Lungs are in balance; if the physiological functions of the Stomach and Lungs and other organs lose this balance, the formation of Qi will be affected. The transportation and transformation functions of the Stomach and Spleen are very important in the process of Qi formation. The nutrients of food and water are the basic substances of the human body in maintaining the vital activities. Through the digestion and absorption of the Spleen and Stomach, food and water can be transformed into the nutrient part to nourish the body; with the nourishment of the nutrient part of the food and water, the congenital Essence can maintain the normal physiological functions.

3. THE PHYSIOLOGICAL FUNCTIONS OF QI

Qi is the fundamental substance in maintaining the vital activities of the human body. Its main physiological functions include the following.

3.1 The promoting function

This refers to the stimulating and promoting effects of Qi. Qi is the very active substance of the Essence: it can stimulate and promote the growth and development of the human body, and the physiological functions of all the Zang Fu organs, meridians and tissues. Qi can also promote the formation and circulation of the Blood, and the formation, distribution and secretion of the Body Fluids; deficiency of Qi can lead to pathological changes such as retarded development of the human body or early aging, even to Blood deficiency, poor circulation of Blood or retention of water and fluids.

3.2 The warming function

Qi is the source of Heat in the human body. The normal temperature of the body is maintained and readjusted by Qi. The normal physiological functions of the Zang Fu organs, meridians and tissues should be maintained at a relatively stable temperature; this temperature is very helpful for the normal circulation of Blood and Body Fluids.

The dysfunction of Qi in warming the body can lead to symptoms such as low body temperature, cold body and cold limbs, or the Cold can transform into Heat, due to the Qi stagnation.

3.3 The protecting function

Qi can protect the body surface and defend it from the invasion of external pathogenic factors. 'Pathogens attack the body only when the Qi is deficient' means that the pathogenic factors attack the body and make the body ill only when the defending function of Qi is weak.

If the defending function of Qi is weak, the body resistance will be reduced and the body gets ill easily.

3.4 The checking function

Qi can check and prevent the Blood, Body Fluid and other fluids from flowing away. It means that the Qi checks and controls the Blood to prevent it from flowing out of the bood vessels; it can also control sweating, urine and nasal discharge, saliva and Stomach fluid, intestine fluid, and sperm.

If the defending function of Qi is weak, a large amount of the Body Fluids will get lost, and symptoms such as bleeding, incontinence, and seminal emission will occur.

The checking and promoting functions of Qi are counteracting and interassisting. Qi promotes the circulation of Blood, and the distribution and secretion of Body Fluids; Qi also checks and controls the fluids in the body and prevents them from flowing away abnormally. These two functions of the Qi work together to maintain the normal circulation, secretion, and discharging of the fluids in the body.

3.5 Qihua (activities of Qi)

Qihua refers to all kinds of changes through the activities of Qi. In detail, it refers to the metabolism and intertransformation of the Essence, Qi, Blood, and Body Fluids. For example, food and water transform into nutrients, and then into the Qi, Blood and Body Fluids; Body Fluids transform into sweat and urine; after digestion and absorption, the food and water can be transformed into wastes in a further step.

The abnormal checking function of the Qi can affect the whole metabolism of the materials and energy. It can affect the digestion and absorption of food and water, then affect the formation and distribution of the Essence, Qi, Blood and Body Fluids, and also the formation and discharge of sweat and urine. In fact, it affects the whole process of body metabolism – the process of the transformation of matter and energy.

4. THE MOVEMENTS OF QI AND THE FORMS OF MOVEMENTS

Mechanism of Qi: Qi movement.

Basic movements of Qi: Ascending, descending, leaving and entering are the four types of Qi movements. Qi moves constantly, and flows all over the body. It promotes and stimulates the physiological functions of the Zang Fu organs, meridians and tissues, as well as the circulation of the Blood and Body Fluids. The balance of the ascending and descending movements are the key point for the Zang Fu organs in maintaining the normal vital activities. For example, in the respiration function of the Lungs, exhalation is the leaving movement of Qi, inhalation is the entering movement of Qi, dispersing is the ascending movement of Qi, and the descending action of Lung-Qi is the descending movement of Qi. They are opposite movements but united in their function. From the general point of view, all physiological activities must be in coordination; looking into various parts of the body, they have their predominant or normal way of movement. For example, the Qi of Liver and Spleen must ascend; Lung and Stomach-Qi descend, when these organs are functioning normally.

The abnormal Qi movements are as follows:

> Qi stagnation → Qi is blocked in a localized area of the body
>
> Reverse flow of Qi → over ascending, less descending of Qi
>
> Sinking of Qi → over descending, less ascending of Qi
>
> Qi collapse → Qi leaves the body, cannot be held inside
>
> Closed Qi → Qi is closed inside, cannot go out

Disharmony of Qi in the Zang Fu organs: For example, Lung-Qi fails in dispersing and descending, the Spleen-Qi sinks down; the Stomach-Qi rebels and goes upward, the Kidneys fail to receive Qi; as a result, Liver-Qi is stagnant.

5. THE DISTRIBUTION AND CLASSIFICATION OF QI

Here we look at the classification of the various types of Qi according to their main constituent parts, distribution, location and special functions.

5.1 Yuan Qi/Primary Qi

This is also called 'Original Qi' or 'Genuine Qi'. It is the most fundamental and important Qi, as well as the primary moving force for the vital activities of the human body.

Formation: Derived from the congenital Essence that is stored in the Kidneys, it needs to be supplemented and nourished by the food and water Essence that is transported and transformed by the Spleen and Stomach. Making use of the Triple Burner as the passage, it can be sent to the Zang Fu organs internally and the body surface externally.

Functions: Promoting the growth and development of the human body, stimulating and promoting the physiological functions of all the Zang Fu organs, meridians and tissues. If Yuan Qi is sufficient, all the Zang Fu organs and related tissues will be active and healthy.

Congenital deficiency of the body, insufficient postnatal nourishment, or prolonged illness, can all lead to a deficiency in Yuan Qi/Primary Qi. When this happens to children they may suffer from retarded growth and development; when it happens to the adults, they may suffer from Qi deficiency of the Zang Fu organs or reduced reproductive function.

5.2 Zong Qi/Pectoral Qi

This is the Qi gathered in the chest. The place where the Zong Qi/Pectoral Qi gathers in the chest is called 'the Sea of Qi' – 'Shanzhong'.

Formation: It is formed by the combination of the Water and food Essence that are transported and transformed by Spleen and Stomach, and the Qing Qi – clear and clean Qi from the air that is inhaled by the Lungs.

Functions:

- It helps the Lungs to control respiration. The strength of speech, voice and respiration are related to the deficiency and excess of Zong Qi/Pectoral Qi. If Zong Qi/Pectoral Qi is sufficient, speech is clear, the voice is strong and respiration is even; if Zong Qi/Pectoral Qi is insufficient, then speech will be unclear, the voice will be feeble and respiration will be weak, even causing asthma.

- It goes along the Heart Meridian and can activate the Blood circulation. The circulation of Blood, the temperature and the activity of the body, the sensations of vision and hearing, and the strength and rhythm of the heartbeat are all related to the condition of Zong Qi/Pectoral Qi.

5.3 Ying Qi/Nutrient Qi

This is also called 'Rong Qi' – 'Ying-nutrient and Blood'. It flows together with Blood in the blood vessels, and is full of nutrition. Compared to the Wei Qi/Defensive Qi, Ying Qi/Nutrient Qi pertains to Yin, and therefore it also has another name 'Ying-nutrient Yin'.

Formation: It is derived from the Essence part of the nutritive food and Water that is produced by the Spleen and Stomach.

Function: To nourish and produce the Blood.

5.4 Wei Qi/Defensive Qi

This flows outside the bood vessels. Compared to Ying Qi/Nutrient Qi, it pertains to Yang, and is also known as 'Defensive Yang'.

Formation: It is derived from water and food Essence. It is characterized as 'fierce and bold'; it is very active, and moves fast; it travels outside the vessels, but between the skin and muscles, moving within the chest and abdominal cavities.

Functions: It protects body surface and defends the body from attack by external pathogens; it warms and nourishes the Zang Fu organs, tissues, skin and body hair. It can also regulate the opening and closing of the body pores, and the secretion of sweat.

5.5 Comparison between Ying Qi/Nutrient Qi and Wei Qi/Defensive Qi

Both of these are derived from water and food Essence, but 'Ying Qi/Nutrient Qi travels inside the vessels and Wei Qi/Defensive Qi travels outside the vessels.' Ying Qi/Nutrient Qi holds itself inside and pertains to Yin, Wei Qi/Defensive Qi defends the outside and pertains to Yang. They work together in coordination to maintain the normal opening and closing of the body pores and the normal body temperature, 'Being active in daytime and sleeping at night', and the normal ability to defend the body from external pathogens. If there is disharmony between Ying Qi/Nutrient Qi and Wei Qi/Defensive Qi, symptoms such as chills and fever, no sweating or profuse sweating, 'Having an unclear mind in daytime and being sleepless at night', and low body resistance may occur.

II. BLOOD

1. THE CONCEPT OF BLOOD

Blood is a red liquid that circulates in the vessels and is full of nutrition. It is the fundamental substance in forming the body and maintaining its vital activities, and has a great function in nourishing and moisturizing the human body.

Vessels: These are the passages within which the Blood circulates, also known as 'Blood House'.

The Blood outside the vessels: On some occasions the Blood flows out of the vessels, which is bleeding.

2. THE FORMATION OF BLOOD

Blood is formed by Ying Qi/Nutrient Qi and Body Fluids. Ying Qi/Nutrient Qi and Body Fluids are derived from the food and water Essence produced by the Spleen and Stomach, and therefore the Spleen and Stomach are known as 'the source of Qi and Blood'. The formation of Blood requires the help of Ying Qi/Nutrient Qi and the Lungs. In addition, the Essence and Blood can be transformed from each other – Essence and Blood share the same source.

Essence and Blood share the same source: Essence is stored in the Kidneys while the Blood is stored in the Liver; sufficient Essence in the Kidneys can nourish the Liver Blood, and sufficient Blood in the Liver can help the Kidneys to store enough Essence, as shown in Figure 3.2.

The Essence stored in the Kidneys	→	Essence, Ying Qi/ Nutrient Qi, Body Fluids	←	Transportation and transformation of Stomach and Spleen, food and water Essence

Figure 3.2

3. THE FUNCTIONS OF BLOOD

To nourish and moisten the whole body: Under the synthesizing functions of the Heart, Lungs, Spleen and Liver, the Blood circulates inside the vessels all over the body and provides the nourishment for all the Zang Fu organs and tissues; the Body Fluids inside the Blood have a moisturizing function. Dysfunction of any of them may cause low body resistance, sallow complexion or a lustreless face, palpitations, dry skin, numbness of the fingers and toes, inflexible movement and a thin pulse.

The fundamental basis for the mental activities: When there is sufficient Blood, smooth Blood circulation and harmonized Zang Fu functions, energy will be vigorous, the Mind will be clear, and sensations will be sharp. However, if the Blood is not sufficient, there will be mental symptoms such as low spirits, being easily frightened, insomnia, dream-disturbed sleep, and poor memory; if Heat enters into the Blood and disturbs the Heart-Mind, mental disorders such as irritability or even coma can result.

4. THE CIRCULATION OF BLOOD

The Blood circulates constantly in the vessels through the entire body and nourishes the Zang Fu organs, tissues, body and limbs continuously.

The circulation of Blood:

- The circulation relies on the pushing function of the Qi. Qi is the motivating source for the circulation of Blood, the reasons for this being: the Heart dominates the Blood and vessels; the Lungs rule the Qi and assist the Heart moving the Blood and the Liver in maintaining the free flow of Qi. If Qi fails to push the Blood, the Blood circulation will slow down and become stagnant.

- The checking function of the Qi can protect the Blood from flowing out of the vessels. The Spleen controls the Blood, and the Liver stores the Blood, and they work together to maintain the normal circulation of the Blood. If the checking function is abnormal, the Blood will flow out of the vessels and lead to bleeding.

III. BODY FLUIDS

1. THE CONCEPT OF BODY FLUIDS

Body Fluids (Jin and Ye): This is a collective term for all the normal fluids of the body. It includes the fluids of the Zang Fu organs and tissues, and their normal secretions, such as stomach fluid, intestinal fluid, nasal discharge, tears and saliva. Body Fluids are the basic substances in forming the body and maintaining the normal vital activities.

The Jin and Ye: Both of these belong to the Body Fluids and are formed from food and drink through the functions of the Spleen and Stomach. Generally speaking, fluid that is thin and clear in nature flows more freely, and distributes to the body surface, skin, muscles and sense organs, penetrates to the bood vessels and has the moistening function, is considered to be Jin; on the other hand, fluid that is thick in nature, with a lower tendency to move, flows into the joints, Zang Fu organs, brain and marrow, and has the nourishment function, is considered to be Ye.

2. THE FORMATION, DISTRIBUTION AND SECRETION OF THE BODY FLUIDS

Body Fluids originate from food and drink after digestion and absorption by the Spleen, Stomach, Small Intestine and Large Intestine. *Plain Questions* states the concept and formation of the Body Fluids as follows:

> After food enters the Stomach, the Qi of food Essence and water is transmitted to the Spleen, Spleen spreads it to the Lungs. The Lungs regulate the water passages and transmits the water to the Bladder below. The Qi and Water then spread in four directions and travel along the meridians of the five Zang organs.

2.1 The formation of the Body Fluids

The food and drink that are digested and absorbed by the Stomach will be continuously separated by the Small Intestine into the clear part and the turbid part, then transported to the Spleen. The distribution and secretion of Body Fluids mainly takes place through the transformation and transportation function of the Spleen, dispersing and descending function of the Lungs, the activities of the Kidneys and the distribution function of the Triple Burner.

2.2 The distribution and secretion of Body Fluids

The distribution of the Body Fluids by the Spleen is described by *Plain Questions* as: 'Spleen moves the Body Fluids for the Stomach.' Through the meridians, the Spleen and Stomach can send out and spread the Body Fluids everywhere in the body; Body Fluids are sent up to the Lungs through the function of the Spleen in spreading the Essence.

The distribution and secretion of the Body Fluids by the Lungs: This is the function of the Lungs in regulating the passage of water. Body Fluids are sent to the whole body surface and nourish the whole body through the dispersing function of the Lungs. Body Fluids will be discharged out of the body in the form of sweat. The Body Fluids are descended by the Lungs, and sent down to the Kidneys and Bladder, then discharged out of the body in the form of urine. In addition, a large amount of the fluids will go out of the body through exhalation.

The Kidneys are the predominant organ in the distribution of Body Fluids:

- The water that is used by the Zang Fu organs will be sent down to the Kidneys; with the evaporation function of the Kidney Yang, the clear part of the fluids is sent upward to the Spleen and Lungs, and distributed to the entire body again. The turbid part of the fluids change into the urine and go into the Bladder.

- In order to promote the distribution of Body Fluids, Kidney Yang is the motivating force for the Stomach to digest and absorb the food Essence, for the Spleen to distribute the Essence, and for the Lungs to regulate the Water passage.

3. THE FUNCTION OF THE BODY FLUIDS

Body Fluids can nourish and moisten the body, and transform into the Blood. The fluid that goes to the body surface can moisten the skin and body hairs; the fluid that flows into the body cavities can moisten and protect the eyes, nose, and mouth; the fluid that penetrates to the bood vessels can nourish and smoothen the vessels and form the Blood; the fluid that enters the internal organs and tissues can nourish and moisten the Zang Fu organs and tissues; the fluid that penetrates the bone can nourish and moisten the bone marrow, spinal cord and the brain.

IV. THE RELATIONSHIPS AMONG QI, BLOOD AND BODY FLUIDS

Qi, Blood, Body Fluids are the fundamental substances in forming the human body and maintaining the vital activities. They cannot exist without the water and food Essence that are transported and transformed by the Spleen and Stomach. They rely on each other, restrain and assist each other, and their pathological changes also affect each other.

1. THE RELATIONSHIP BETWEEN QI AND BLOOD

Qi pertains to Yang while the Blood pertains to Yin. Qi is considered to be the governor of Blood, and Blood is the mother of Qi.

1.1 Qi produces Blood

The formation and production of Blood cannot occur without Qi and Qi activities.

- Ying Qi/Nutrient Qi is directly involved in the formation of Blood, and this is the main part of the Blood.

- The activities of Qi are the motivating force for producing the Blood. It is very important in the whole process through which the body takes in food and water, changing them into Essence, and transforming them into the Ying Qi/Nutrient Qi, Body Fluids and Blood.

1.2 Qi moves the Blood

Blood pertains to Yin and is considered a quiet substance. Blood cannot move without the pushing of Qi. Qi moves Blood, and disturbance of Qi movement will lead to the stagnation of Blood. The circulation of Blood needs the pushing of Heart-Qi, dispersing of Lung-Qi, and free flowing of Liver-Qi. Therefore, a deficiency of Qi may cause a reduction in the pushing function of Qi; stagnation of Qi may cause the Blood to flow slowly, even to stagnate; a disorder of the movement of Qi may lead the Blood to flow in the wrong direction: there will be symptoms such as a red face and eyes, headache, and vomiting of Blood if the Blood goes up with the Qi moving upward; if the Blood flows down while the Qi is sinking epigastric and abdominal distention, vaginal bleeding and dysfunctional uterine bleeding.

1.3 Qi controls the Blood

Qi can control the Blood so that it circulates within the vessels instead of going out of the vessels. In fact, this refers specifically to the function of Spleen-Qi in controlling the Blood.

The above mentioned three aspects can be summarized as 'Qi is the governor of the Blood'.

1.4 Blood is the mother of Qi

Blood is the carrier of Qi, and it provides sufficient nutrition for Qi. Qi must connect with the Blood and Body Fluids in order to stay within the body. If Qi loses its carrier, it will lose its root and become collapsed. If Blood is deficient, Qi will become weak easily; if Blood becomes collapsed, Qi also collapses easily. In the treatment of severe bleeding, the method of reinforcing Qi in order to control the loss of Blood can be applied.

2. THE RELATIONSHIP BETWEEN QI AND BODY FLUIDS

The formation, distribution and secretion of the Body Fluids rely on the ascending, descending, leaving and entering movements of the Qi, and the Qi activities – the warming, pushing and checking functions of the Qi. Qi exists inside the body and connects with the Blood and Body Fluids, and the Body Fluids are the carrier for Qi.

2.1 Qi produces Body Fluids

The formation of the Body Fluids depends on the function of the Stomach in digesting and absorbing food and water, and the function of the Spleen in transforming and transporting the food and water Essence. Strong and sufficient Spleen and Stomach-Qi can produce sufficient Body Fluids; weak and deficient Qi can lead to the lack of production of Body Fluids.

2.2 Qi moves the Body Fluids

Qi is the motivating force for the to distribution and secretion of the Body Fluids. The ascending, descending, leaving and entering movements of Qi can help to distribute the Body Fluids all over the body, and discharge them out of the body as urine and sweat. Through the transforming and transporting function of the Spleen, the dispersing and descending function of the Lungs, and the evaporation function of the Kidneys, the Body Fluids can be sent to the entire body; through metabolism, the Body Fluids will be discharged as sweat and urine. If Qi movement is abnormal, the distribution of the Body Fluids will also be affected, the obstruction of the Body Fluids may result, and then the ascending, descending, leaving and entering of the Qi will function abnormally as well. Qi deficiency or Qi stagnation can lead to the obstruction of fluids, described as 'Qi fails in moving the water'; the retention of Body Fluids can lead to the disorder of Qi movement, described as 'retained water causes Qi stagnation'. The activities of Qi and Body Fluids are both the causes and consequences of each other's condition, and the pathological results are the retention of Water, Phlegm and Dampness, or oedema.

2.3 Qi checks Body Fluids, and Body Fluids carry the Qi

The secretion of the Body Fluids relies on the promoting activities of Qi. The checking function of Qi is also important in order to prevent the Body Fluids from flowing away abnormally. If Qi is deficient or the checking function is reduced, the Body Fluids will be lost abnormally, and pathological changes such as profuse sweating, profuse urination, or enuresis can be seen; on the other hand, Body Fluids are the carriers of Qi: if large amounts of fluids are lost through profuse sweating, profuse urination, vomiting and diarrhoea, then diseases such as Qi collapse, with the collapse of the Body Fluids, can occur.

3. THE RELATIONSHIP BETWEEN BLOOD AND BODY FLUIDS

Both Blood and Body Fluids are liquids, and have moistening and nourishing functions. They both originate from food and water Essence, and therefore 'They share the same source'. Body Fluids enter the vessels and become a part of the Blood. Blood and Body Fluids not only transform into each other and assist each other, but also pathologically affect each other. If there is too much bleeding, Body Fluids outside the vessels will enter the vessels to reinforce the Blood and then the Body Fluids outside the vessels will become deficient, with symptoms such as thirst, scanty urine, and dry skin; if a large amount of the Body Fluids is consumed, the Body Fluids in the vessels will flow out, and then there will be problems such as deficiency of Blood, shortage of fluids and Dryness of Blood. For those reasons, to treat a bleeding patient, the 'promoting sweat' method should be avoided. In *Treatise On Exogenous Febrile Diseases* it is stated: 'The perspiring method should not be used for nasal bleeding patient.' For the patient who loses a large amount of Body Fluids through sweating, or has a severe deficiency of Body Fluids, a strong herbal formula to break Blood stagnation or remove the stagnant Blood should be carefully used. As mentioned in *Miraculous Pivot*: 'The patient who loses Blood should avoid perspiring while the patient who sweats a lot should avoid losing Blood,' which is the basis for the application of the theory 'Body Fluids and Blood share the same source' in the clinic.

MERIDIANS AND COLLATERALS

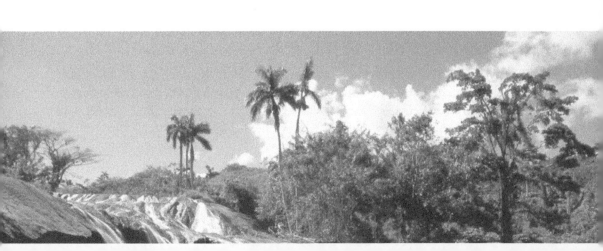

I. BRIEF INTRODUCTION

MERIDIAN THEORY

This is one of the important theories of Traditional Chinese Medicine, which includes the physiology and pathology of the meridian system and its relationship with the Zang Fu organs, and which was systematized by the ancient Chinese people in their prolonged clinical practice. This theory was formed when ancient people used stone needles, conduction exercises (ancient deep breathing exercises), massage and Qigong as therapies and health-care approaches. It is based on the transmission of needling sensation, ancient anatomical knowledge and philosophy.

II. THE CONCEPT OF THE MERIDIANS AND COLLATERALS AND THEIR COMPOSITION

1. THE CONCEPT OF THE MERIDIANS AND COLLATERALS

The meridians and collaterals: These are pathways in which the Qi and Blood of the human body circulate. They pertain to the Zang Fu organs in the interior of the body and extend over the body to the exterior, linking the tissues into an organic whole.

The meridians: These constitute the main trunks, and run longitudinally. They each have their fixed courses.

The collaterals: These represent branches of the meridians and run transversely.
   The meridians and collaterals closely connect with each other, connecting the organs and tissues into an organic whole.

2. THE COMPOSITION OF THE MERIDIANS AND COLLATERALS

The system of the meridians and collaterals includes: the twelve main meridians, eight extra meridians, twelve divergent meridians, fifteen collaterals, twelve muscle regions and twelve cutaneous regions (see Figure 4.1). Internally they connect with the Zang Fu organs and externally with the muscles and skin.

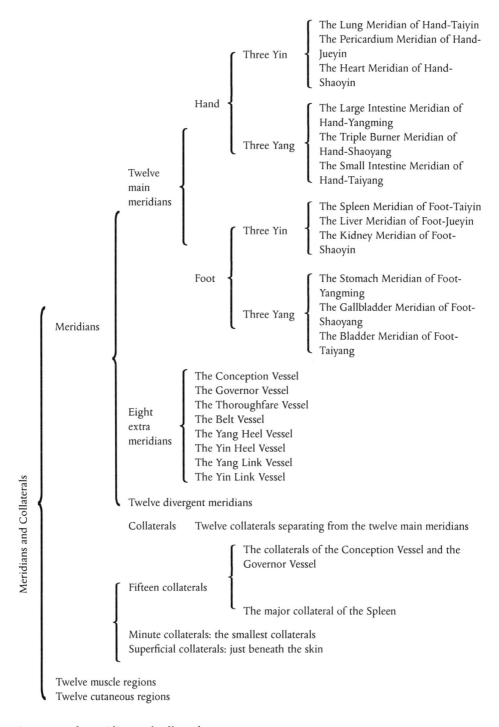

Figure 4.1: The meridians and collaterals

2.1 The twelve main meridians

The twelve main meridians include: the three Yin meridians of the hand, the three Yin meridians of the foot, the three Yang meridians of the hand and the three Yang meridians of the foot. They are distributed symmetrically on the left and right sides of the body. Directly pertaining to the Zang Fu organs, the twelve main meridians each have their fixed courses, specific order of the cyclic flow of Qi and Blood, and rules whereby they run through their courses.

2.2 The eight extra meridians

These are the Governor Vessel, Conception Vessel, Thoroughfare Vessel, Belt Vessel, Yang Heel Vessel, Yin Heel Vessel, Yang Link Vessel and Yin Link Vessel. The eight extra meridians assume the responsibility of controlling, joining and regulating the twelve main meridians.

2.3 The twelve divergent meridians

The twelve divergent meridians branch out from the twelve main meridians. They derive from the main meridians in the regions of the four limbs, then enter the thoracic and abdominal cavities and, at last, emerge at the neck. Their function is to strengthen the relationship between the internally–externally related meridians. They also supplement the pathway that the main meridians do not reach.

2.4 The fifteen collaterals

These separate from the twelve main meridians, including minute collaterals and superficial collaterals. Minute collaterals are the smallest collaterals. Superficial collaterals lie just beneath the skin. The fifteen collaterals include the twelve collaterals separating from the twelve main meridians, the collaterals of the Conception Vessel and Governor Vessel and the major collateral of the Spleen. Their function is to strengthen the superficial connection between the externally–internally related meridians.

2.5 The twelve muscle regions and twelve cutaneous regions

The muscle regions refer to the muscle system and skin relating to the twelve main meridians. They are the sites where the Qi of the twelve main meridians starts, knots, gathers and spreads in the muscles and joints. The functions of the muscle regions are to connect the bones of the skeleton and maintain movement of the joints.

The cutaneous regions are twelve distinct areas on the body surface within the domains of the twelve main meridians. These areas respond to the function of the twelve main meridians.

3. THE FUNCTIONS OF THE MERIDIANS AND COLLATERALS

These are:

- circulating Qi and Blood, balancing Yin and Yang

- resisting pathogens and protecting the body

- transmitting needling sensations and regulating deficiency and excess conditions.

III. THE TWELVE MAIN MERIDIANS

1. THE NOMENCLATURE OF THE TWELVE MAIN MERIDIANS

These are distributed symmetrically on the left and right sides of the body. Yin and Yang meridians are named according to the aspect of the four limbs – namely, Yin aspect (medial side) or Yang aspect (lateral side), along which runs the meridian. Yin meridians can be divided into Taiyin, Jueyin and Shaoyin; while Yang merdians can be divided into Yangming, Shaoyang and Taiyang. The meridians are named according to their connecting organs, so hand or foot (at which their point begins or terminates), Yin or Yang, Zang or Fu are the three components in the nomenclature of the meridian names.

Nomenclature of the twelve main meridians

	Yin meridian (pertains to Zang organ)	Yang meridian (pertains to Fu organ)	Distribution (Yang meridian at the lateral side, Yin meridian at the medial side)	
Hand	The Lung Meridian of Hand-Taiyin	The Large Intestine Meridian of Hand-Yangming	*Upper limb*	Anterior
	The Pericardium Meridian of Hand-Jueyin	The Triple Burner Meridian of Hand-Shaoyang		Intermediate
	The Heart Meridian of Hand-Shaoyin	The Small Intestine Meridian of Hand-Taiyang		Posterior
Foot	The Spleen Meridian of Foot-Taiyin	The Stomach Meridian of Foot-Yangming	*Lower limb*	Anterior
	The Liver Meridian of Foot-Jueyin	The Gallbladder Meridian of Foot-Shaoyang		Intermediate
	The Kidney Meridian of Foot-Shaoyin	The Bladder Meridian of Foot-Taiyang		Posterior

2. THE REGULATION OF THE RUNNING COURSES AND CYCLICAL FLOW OF QI

The three Yin meridians of the hand run from the chest to the hand; the three Yang meridians of the hand run from the hand to the head; the three Yang meridians of the foot run from the head to the foot; and the three Yin meridians of the foot run from the foot to the abdomen. The Yin and Yang meridians are connected with each other, forming an continuous circulation of Yin–Yang.

3. DISTRIBUTION

3.1 On the limbs

Here the medial aspects are supplied by the three Yin meridians, while the lateral aspects are supplied by the three Yang meridians, as shown in the following table.

Distribution of the meridians in the limbs

Location		Area supplied	
		Medial (Yin meridian)	**Lateral (Yang meridian)**
Upper limb	Anterior	Hand-Taiyin Meridian	Hand-Yangming Meridian
	Intermediate	Hand-Jueyin Meridian	Hand-Shaoyang Meridian
	Posterior	Hand-Shaoyin Meridian	Hand-Taiyang Meridian
Lower limb	Anterior	Foot-Taiyin Meridian	Foot-Yangming Meridian
	Intermediate	Foot-Jueyin Meridian	Foot-Shaoyang Meridian
	Posterior	Foot-Shaoyin Meridian	Foot-Taiyang Meridian

The crossing point of the Spleen Meridian and Liver Meridian is situated 8 cun superior to the medial malleolus. Below this point, the Liver Meridian goes in front of the Spleen Meridian, and above this point, it goes behind the Spleen Meridian.

3.2 On the head and face

The Yangming Meridians run in the facial and frontal regions; the Taiyang Meridians run in the cheek, vertex and occiput; the Shaoyang Meridians travel in the lateral aspects of the head. The Jueyin Meridian of Foot also runs to the vertex.

Distribution of the meridians in the head

	Location	Distribution of meridian
Anterior	Front	Hand-Yangming
	Cheek	Hand-Taiyang
Lateral	Temple	Hand-Shaoyang
Posterior	Vertex, occiput	Foot-Taiyang

3.3 In the trunk

The three Yang meridians of the hand run along the scapula (shoulder blade) region. The three Yin meridians of the hand emerge from the axillary (the armpit). The Yangming Meridian of Foot runs over the anterior aspect (chest and abdomen). The Taiyang Meridian of Foot runs over the posterior aspect (back). The Shaoyang Meridian of Foot runs along the lateral side. The three Yin meridians of the foot go along the abdomen – details are shown in the table that follows.

Distribution of meridians in the trunk

Location		The first lateral line	The second lateral line	The third lateral line
Anterior	Chest	The Kidney Meridian (2 cun lateral to the anterior midline)	The Stomach Meridian (4 cun lateral to the anterior midline)	The Spleen Meridian (6 cun lateral to the anterior midline)
	Abdomen	The Kidney Meridian (0.5 cun lateral to the anterior midline)	The Stomach Meridian (2 cun lateral to the anterior midline)	The Spleen Meridian (4 cun lateral to the anterior midline)
Posterior	Back and low back	The Bladder Meridian (1.5 cun lateral to the posterior midline)	The Bladder Meridian (3 cun lateral to the posterior midline)	The Liver Meridian (ascends obliquely from the lower abdomen to the hypochondriac region)
	Scapula (shoulderblade)	Three Yang meridians of the hand		
Lateral	Axilla (armpit)	Three Yin meridians of the hand		
	Hypochondriac region, lateral side of the abdomen	The Gallbladder Meridian, the Liver Meridian		

The Distribution of meridian spans the three lateral line columns.

4. THE CYCLICAL FLOW OF QI IN THE TWELVE MAIN MERIDIANS

The twelve main meridians are distributed in different parts of the body. The cyclical flow of Qi and Blood in the meridians starts from the Lung Meridian of Hand-Taiyin, and ends up with the Liver Meridian of Foot-Jueyin, then runs back to the Lung Meridian of Hand-Taiyin. The twelve main meridians link to one another in a fixed order. A cyclical flow of Qi is thus maintained by their mutual connection.

The Lung Meridian of Hand-Taiyin → The Large Intestine Meridian of Hand-Yangming → The Stomach Meridian of Foot-Yangming → The Spleen Meridian of Foot-Taiyin → The Heart Meridian of Hand-Shaoyin → The Small Intestine Meridian of Hand-Taiyang → The Bladder Meridian of Foot-Taiyang → The Kidney Meridian of Foot-Shaoyin → The Pericardium Meridian of Hand-Jueyin → The Triple Burner Meridian of Hand-Shaoyang →The Gallbladder Meridian of Foot-Shaoyang → The Liver Meridian of Foot-Jueyin

5. EXTERIOR-INTERIOR RELATIONSHIPS

The Yin meridians and Yang meridians are connected by the divergent meridians and collaterals, forming six paired exterior–interior relationships.

The six paired exterior–interior relationships

Exterior	Hand-Yangming	Hand-Shaoyang	Hand-Taiyang	Foot-Yangming	Foot-Shaoyang	Foot-Taiyang
Interior	Hand-Taiyin	Hand-Jueyin	Hand-Shaoyin	Foot-Taiyin	Foot-Jueyin	Foot-Shaoyin

The exterior–interior relationship of the meridians is strengthened by the confluence of the two coupled meridians. As the two coupled meridians pertain to the same pair of Zang Fu organs, this pair of organs has physiological and pathological influences upon each other. In practice, the points of the externally–internally related meridians can be used interchangeably, for example, points of the Liver Meridian are used for treating Gallbladder disorders.

6. THE COURSES OF THE TWELVE MAIN MERIDIANS

6.1 The Lung Meridian of Hand-Taiyin

The Lung Meridian of Hand-Taiyin starts from the Middle Burner, and descends to connect with the Large Intestine. Winding back, it goes up the diaphragm, and links with the Lungs. From the Lung system, which refers to the portion of the Lung communicating with the throat, it comes out transversely (Zhongfu, LU1). Descending along the medial aspect of the upper arm, it passes in front of the Heart Meridian of Hand-Shaoyin and the Pericardium Meridian of Hand-Jueyin, and reaches the cubital fossa. Then it goes continuously downward along the anterior border of the radial side in the medial aspect of the forearm and enters Cunkou. Passing the thenar eminence, it goes along its radial border, ending at the medial side of the tip of the thumb (Shaoshang, LU11).

The branch proximal to the wrist emerges from Lieque (LU7) and runs directly to the radial side of the tip of the index finger (Shangyang, LI1) where it links with the Large Intestine Meridian of Hand-Yangming.

6.2 The Large Intestine Meridian of Hand-Yangming

The Large Intestine Meridian of Hand-Yangming starts from the tip of the index finger (Shangyang, LI1). Running upward along the radial side of the index finger and passing through the interspace of the first and second metacarpal bones, it then enters the depression between the tendons of m.extensor pollicis longus and brevis. Then, following the lateral anterior aspect of the forearm, it reaches the lateral side of the elbow. From there, it ascends along the lateral anterior aspect of the upper arm to the highest point of the shoulder (Jianyu, LI15). Then, along the anterior border of the acromion, it goes up to the seventh cervical vertebra (the confluence of the three Yang meridians of the hand and foot) (Dazhui, GV14), and descends to the supraclavicular fossa to connect with the Lungs. It then passes through the diaphragm and enters the Large Intestine, the organ to which it pertains.

The branch from the supraclavicular fossa runs upward to the neck, passes through the cheek and enters the gums of the lower teeth. Then it curves around the upper lip and crosses the opposite meridian at the philtrum. From there, the left meridian goes to the right and the right meridian to the left, to both sides of the nose (Yingxiang, LI20), where the Large Intestine Meridian links with the Stomach Meridian of Foot-Yangming.

6.3 The Stomach Meridian of Foot-Yangming

The Stomach Meridian of Foot-Yangming starts from the side of the nostril (Yingxiang, LI20). It ascends to the bridge of the nose, where it meets the Bladder Meridian of Foot-Taiyang (Jingming, BL1). Turning downward along the lateral side of nose (Chengqi, ST1), it enters the upper gum. Reemerging, it curves around the lips and descends to meet the Conception Vessel at the mentolabial groove (Chengjiang, CV24). Then it runs postero-laterally across the lower portion of the cheek at Daying (ST5). Winding along the angle of the mandible (Jiache, ST6), it ascends in front of the ear and traverses Shangguan (GB3). Then it follows the anterior hairline and reaches the forehead. The facial branch emerging in front of Daying (ST5) runs downward to Renying (ST9). From there it goes along the throat and enters the supraclavicular fossa. Descending, it passes through the diaphragm, enters the Stomach, its pertaining organ, and connects with the Spleen.

The straight portion of the meridian arising from the supraclavicular fossa runs downward, passing through the nipple. It descends by the umbilicus and enters Qichong (ST30) on the lateral side of the lower abdomen.

The branch from the lower orifice of the Stomach descends inside the abdomen and joins the previous portion of the meridian at Qichong (ST30). Running downward traversing Biguan (ST31), and further through Femur-Futu (ST32), it reaches the knee. From there, it continues downward along the anterior border of the lateral aspect of the tibia, passes through the dorsum of the foot, and reaches the lateral side of the tip of the second toe (Lidui, ST45).

The tibial branch emerges from Zusanli (ST36), 3 cun below the knee, and enters the lateral side of the middle toe.

The branch from the dorsum of the foot arises from Chongyang (ST42) and terminates at the medial side of the tip of the great toe (Yinbai, SP1), where it links with the Spleen Meridian of Foot-Taiyin.

6.4 The Spleen Meridian of Foot-Taiyin

The Spleen Meridian of Foot-Taiyin starts from the tip of the big toe (Yinbai, SP1). It runs along the medial aspect of the foot at the junction of the red and white skin, and ascends in front of the medial malleolus up to the medial aspect of the leg. It follows the posterior aspect of the tibia, crosses and goes in front of the Liver Meridian of Foot-Jueyin. Passing through the anterior medial aspect of the knee and thigh, it enters the abdomen, then the Spleen, its pertaining organ, and connects with the Stomach. From there it ascends, passing through the diaphragm and running alongside the oesophagus. When it reaches the root of the tongue it spreads over its lower surface.

The branch from the Stomach goes upward through the diaphragm, and flows into the Heart to link with the Heart Meridian of Hand-Shaoyin.

6.5 The Heart Meridian of Hand-Shaoyin

The Heart Meridian of Hand-Shaoyin originates from the Heart. Emerging, it spreads over the 'Heart system' (i.e. the tissues connecting the Heart with the other Zang Fu organs). It passes through the diaphragm to connect with the Small Intestine.

The ascending portion of the meridian from the 'Heart system' runs alongside the oesophagus to connect with the 'eye system' (i.e. the tissues connecting the eyes with the brain).

The straight portion of the meridian from the 'Heart system' goes upward to the Lungs. Then it turns downward and emerges from the axilla (Jiquan, HT1). From there it goes along the posterior border of the medial aspect of the upper arm behind the Lung Meridian of Hand-Taiyin and the Pericardium Meridian of Hand-Jueyin down to the cubital fossa. From there it descends along the posterior border of the medial aspect of the forearm to the pisiform region proximal to the palm and enters the palm. Then it follows the medial aspect of the little finger to its tip (Shaochong, HT9) and links with the Small Intestine Meridian of Hand-Taiyang.

6.6 The Small Intestine Meridian of Hand-Taiyang

The Small Intestine Meridian of Hand-Taiyang starts from the ulnar side of the tip of the little finger (Shaoze, SI1). Following the ulnar side of the dorsum of the hand it reaches the wrist where it emerges from the styloid process of the ulna. From there it ascends along the posterior aspect of the forearm, passes between the olecranon of the ulna and the medial epicondyle of the humerus, and runs along the posterior border of the lateral aspect of the upper arm to the shoulder joint. Circling around the scapular region, it meets Dazhui (GV14) on the superior aspect of the shoulder. Then, turning downward to the supraclavicular fossa, it connects with the Heart. From there it descends along the oesophagus, passes through the diaphragm, reaches the Stomach, and finally enters the Small Intestine, its pertaining organ.

The branch from the supraclavicular fossa ascends to the neck, and further to the cheek. Via the outer canthus, it enters the ear (Tinggong, SI19).

The branch from the neck runs upward to the infraorbital region (Quanliao, SI18) and further to the lateral side of the nose. Then it reaches the inner canthus (Jingming, BL1) to link with the Bladder Meridian of Foot-Taiyang.

6.7 The Bladder Meridian of Foot-Taiyang

The Bladder Meridian of Foot-Taiyang starts from the inner canthus (Jingming, BL1). Ascending to the forehead, it joins the Governor Vessel at the vertex (Baihui, GV20), where a branch arises, running to the temple.

The straight portion of the meridian enters and communicates with the brian from the vertex. It then emerges and bifurcates to descend along the posterior aspect of the neck. Running downward alongside the medial aspect of the scapular region and parallel to the vertebral column, it reaches the lumbar region, where it enters the body cavity via the paravertebral muscle to connect with the Kidneys and join its pertaining organ, the Bladder.

The branch of the lumbar region descends through the gluteal region and ends in the popliteal fossa.

The branch from the posterior aspect of the neck runs straight downward along the medial border of the scapula. Passing through the gluteal region (Huantiao, GB30) downward along the lateral aspect of the thigh, it meets the preceding branch descending from the lumbar region in the popliteal fossa. From there it descends to the leg and further to the posterior aspect of the external malleolus. Then, running along the tuberosity of the fifth metatarsal bone, it reaches the lateral side of the tip of the little toe (Zhiyin, BL67), where it links with the Kidney Meridian of Foot-Shaoyin.

6.8 The Kidney Meridian of Foot-Shaoyin

The Kidney Meridian of Foot-Shaoyin starts from the inferior aspect of the small toe and runs obliquely towards the sole of the foot (Yongquan, KI1). Emerging from the lower aspect of the tuberosity of the navicular bone and running behind the medial malleolus, it enters the heel. Then it ascends along the medial side of the leg to the medial side of the popliteal fossa and goes further upward along the posteromedial aspect of the thigh towards the vertebral column (Changqiang, GV1), where it enters the Kidneys, its pertaining organ, and connects with the Bladder.

The straight portion of the meridian reemerges from the Kidneys. Ascending and passing through the Liver and diaphragm, it enters the Lungs, runs along the throat and terminates at the root of the tongue.

A branch springs from the Lungs, joins the Heart and runs into the chest to link with the Pericardium Meridian of Hand-Jueyin.

6.9 The Pericardium Meridian of Hand-Jueyin

The Pericardium Meridian of Hand-Jueyin originates from the chest. Emerging, it enters its pertaining organ, the Pericardium. Then, it descends through the diaphragm to the abdomen, connecting successively with the Upper, Middle and Lower Burners.

A branch arising from the chest runs inside the chest, emerges from the costal region at a point 3 cun below the anterior axillary fold (Tianchi, PC1) and ascends to the axilla. Following the medial aspect of the upper arm, it runs downward between the Lung Meridian of Hand-Taiyin and the Heart Meridian of Hand-Shaoyin to the cubital fossa, further downward to the forearm between the two tendons (the tendons of *m. palmaris longus* and *m. flexor carpi radialis*), ending in the palm. From there it passes along the middle finger right down to its tip (Zhongchong, PC9).

Another branch arises from the palm at Laogong (PC8), runs along the ring finger to its tip (Guanchong, TE1) and links with the Triple Burner Meridian of Hand-Shaoyang.

6.10 The Triple Burner Meridian of Hand-Shaoyang

The Triple Burner Meridian of Hand-Shaoyang originates from the tip of the ring finger (Guanchong, TE1), running upward between the fourth and fifth metacarpal bones along the dorsal aspect of the wrist to the lateral aspect of the forearm between the radius and ulna. Passing through the olecranon and along the lateral aspect of the upper arm, it reaches the shoulder region, where it goes across and passes behind the Gallbladder Meridian of Foot-Shaoyang. Winding over to the supraclavicular fossa, it spreads in the chest to connect with the Pericardium. It then descends through the diaphragm down to the abdomen, and joins its pertaining organ, the Upper, Middle and Lower Burner.

A branch originates from the chest. Running upward, it emerges from the supraclavicular fossa. From there it ascends to the neck, running along the posterior border of the ear, and further to the corner of the anterior hairline. Then it turns downward to the cheek and terminates in the infraorbital region.

The auricular branch arises from the retroauricular region and enters the ear. Then it emerges in front of the ear, crosses the previous branch at the cheek and reaches the outer canthus (Sizhukong, TE23) to link with the Gallbladder Meridian of Foot-Shaoyang.

6.11 The Gallbladder Meridian of Foot-Shaoyang

The Gallbladder Meridian of Foot-Shaoyang originates from the outer canthus (Tongziliao, GB1), ascends to the corner of the forehead (Hanyan, GB4), then curves downward to the retroauricular region (Fengchi, GB20) and runs along the side of the neck in front of the Triple Burner Meridian of Hand-Shaoyang to the shoulder. Turning back, it traverses and passes behind the Triple Burner Meridian of Hand-Shaoyang down to the supraclavicular fossa.

The retroauricular branch arises from the retroauricular region and enters the ear. It then comes out and passes the preauricular region to the posterior aspect of the outer canthus.

The branch arising from the outer canthus runs downward to Daying (ST5) and meets the Triple Burner Meridian of Hand-Shaoyang in the infraorbital region. Then, passing through Jiache (ST6), it descends to the neck and enters the supraclavicular fossa where it meets the main meridian. From there it further descends into the chest, passes through the diaphragm to connect with the Liver and enters its pertaining organ, the Gallbladder. Then it runs inside the hypochondriac region, comes out from the lateral side of the lower abdomen near the femoral artery at the inguinal region. From there it runs superficially along the margin of the pubic hair and goes transversely into the hip region (Huantiao, GB30).

The straight portion of the channel runs downward from the supraclavicular fossa, passes in front of the axilla along the lateral aspect of the chest and through the free ends of the floating ribs to the hip region where it meets the previous branch. Then it descends along the lateral aspect of the thigh to the lateral side of the knee. Going further downward along the anterior aspect of the fibula all the way to its lower end (Xuanzhong, GB39), it reaches the anterior aspect of the external malleolus. It then follows the dorsum of the foot to the lateral side of the tip of the fourth toe (Zuqiaoyin, GB44).

The branch of the dorsum of the foot springs from Zulinqi (GB41), runs between the first and second metatarsal bones to the distal portion of the great toe and terminates at its hairy region (Dadun, LR1), where it links with the Liver Meridian of Foot-Jueyin.

6.12 The Liver Meridian of Foot-Jueyin

The Liver Meridian of Foot-Jueyin starts from the dorsal hairy region of the great toe (Dadun, LR1). Running upward along the dorsum of the foot, passing through Zhongfeng (LR4), 1 cun in front of the medial malleolus, it ascends to an area 8 cun above the medial malleolus, where it runs across and behind the Spleen Meridian of Foot-Taiyin. Then it runs further upward to the medial side of the knee and along the medial aspect of the thigh to the pubic hair region, where it curves around the external genitalia and goes up to the lower abdomen. It then runs upward and curves around the Stomach to enter the Liver, its pertaining organ, and connects with the Gallbladder. From there it continues to ascend, passing through the diaphragm, and branching out in the costal and hypochondriac region. Then it ascends along the posterior aspect of the throat to the nasopharynx and connects with the 'eye system'. Running further upward, it emerges from the forehead and meets the Governor Vessel at the vertex.

The branch that arises from the 'eye system' runs downward into the cheek and curves around the inner surface of the lips.

The branch arising from the Liver passes through the diaphragm, runs into the Lungs and links with the Lung Meridian of Hand-Taiyin.

IV. THE EIGHT EXTRA MERIDIANS

1. CONCEPT

The eight extra meridians are the Governor Vessel, the Conception Vessel, the Thoroughfare Vessel, the Belt Vessel, the Yin Heel Vessel, the Yang Heel Vessel, the Yin Link Vessel and the Yang Link Vessel. Their courses of distributions are different from those of the twelve regular meridians and they do not pertain to, or connect with, the Zang Fu organs. But there is a close relationship between the eight extra meridians and the Extraordinary Fu Organs. There is no internal–external relation among the eight extra meridians – and that is why they are called extra meridians.

2. FUNCTION

The extra meridians cross between the twelve regular meridians to enhance the connections of the twelve regular meridians and regulate their Qi and Blood. They are closely related to the Zang organs, such as the Liver and Kidneys, as well as the Extraordinary Fu organs.

3. THE GOVERNOR VESSEL

3.1 Running course

This originates from the inside of the lower abdomen. Descending, it emerges at the perineum. Then it ascends posteriorly along the interior of the spinal column to Fengfu (GV16) at the nape, where it enters and connects the brain. It further ascends along the neck and mid-line of the head, through the forehead, nose, and upper lip to the frenulum of the upper lip (Yinjiao, GV28).

A branch arises from the posterior of the spinal column and connects to the Kidneys. A branch ascends from the interior of the lower abdomen, through the umbilicus, upward to the Heart, the throat and the mandible region. It further curves around the lips and ascends to the middle between the inferior side of the two eyes.

3.2 Function

The Governor Vessel runs in the middle of the back. It meets the six Yang meridians at Dazhui (GV14) and also the Yang Link Vessel. It regulates and governs the Yang meridians of the whole body and is called the 'Sea of the Yang Meridians'. It runs in the posterior of the spinal column and ascends to enter and connect to the brain. A branch arises from the posterior of the spinal column and connects to the Kidneys. So the Governor Vessel has a close relationship with the brain, spinal cord and Kidneys.

4. THE CONCEPTION VESSEL

4.1 Running course

This originates from the inside of the lower abdomen and emerges from the perineum. It runs anteriorly to the pubic region and ascends along the midline of the abdomen and chest to the throat. Running further upward to the mandible, it curves around the lips, passes through the cheek and enters the infraorbital region.

A branch arises from the inside of the lower abdomen and runs posteriorly inside the back.

4.2 Function

The Conception Vessel runs along the midline of the abdomen and meets repeatedly the three Yin meridians of the hand or foot and the Yin Link Meridian. It controls the Yin meridians of the whole body and is called the 'Sea of the Yin Meridians'. It originates from the inside of the lower abdomen and is related to pregnancy, and is therefore described as the 'Conception Vessel Dominating Pregnancy'.

5. THE THOROUGHFARE VESSEL

5.1 Running course

This originates from the inside of the lower abdomen, descends and emerges from the perineum. It then ascends and passes the region of Qichong (ST30), where it coincides with the Kidney Meridian of Foot-Shaoyin. It runs upward along both sides of abdomen to the chest and throat and curves around the lips until it goes into the infraorbital region.

A branch arises from Qichong (ST30) and runs along the medial of the thigh to the popliteal fossa. It then descends along the medial border of the tibia to the sole. Another branch arises from the posterior of the medial malleolus, runs anteriorly and obliquely to the dorsum of foot and enters the big toe.

5.2 Function

The Thoroughfare Vessel ascends to the head and also descends to the foot, running through the whole body. It connects the twelve regular meridians and works as a communications centre to guide the Qi and Blood of various meridians. When there is excess or insufficiency of Qi and Blood in the Zang Fu organs or meridians, the Thoroughfare Meridian may regulate it correspondingly. It is called both the 'Sea of the Twelve Regular Meridians' and the 'Sea of Blood', which indicates its close relation with menstruation.

6. THE BELT VESSEL

6.1 Running course

This starts below the hypochondriac region. Running downward through Daimai (GB26), it descends to the lower abdomen and runs transversely around the waist like a belt.

6.2 Function

The Belt Vessel runs transversely around the waist like a belt in order to restrain the meridians that run longitudinally.

7. THE YIN HEEL AND YANG HEEL VESSELS

7.1 Running course

These are distributed symmetrically on the right and left sides of the body. Both the Yin Heel and Yang Heel Vessels start from the inferior of the malleolus. The Yin Heel Vessel starts from the inferior of the medial malleolus (Zhaohai, KI6). It ascends along the posterior of the medial malleolus in a straight line to the medial aspect of the lower limb. It passes the external genitalia and ascends further along the abdomen and chest to the supraclavicular fossa. Running upward in front of Renying (ST9), it passes the lateral side of the nose to the inner canthus and communicates with the Hand and Foot-Taiyang Meridians and the Yang Heel Vessel.

The Yang Heel Vessel starts from the inferior of the external malleolus (Shenmai, BL62). Ascending along the posterior of the external malleolus, it passes the abdomen, the lateroposterior of the chest, the shoulder, and the lateral of the neck and ascends to the corner of the mouth. Then it enters the inner canthus and communicates with the Hand and Foot-Taiyang Meridians and the Yin Heel Vessel. It then ascends through the hairline and descends to the retroauricular region and meets the Gall Bladder Meridian of Foot-Shaoyang at the posterior of the neck.

7.2 Function

The Yin Heel and Yang Heel Meridians can moisten the eyes and dominate the opening and closing of eyelids as well as the movement of the lower limbs.

8. THE YIN LINK AND YANG LINK VESSELS

8.1 Running course

The Yin Link Vessel starts from the medial side of the leg where the three Yin meridians of the foot meet, and ascends along the medial aspect of the thigh to the abdomen to communicate with the Spleen Meridian of Foot-Taiyin. Then it communicates with the Liver Meridian of Foot-Jueyin and ascends to the throat. There it communicates with the Conception Vessel and terminates at Lianquan (CV23).

The Yang Link Vessel starts from the inferior of the external malleolus and runs upward along the Gallbladder Meridian of Foot-Shaoyang. It then ascends along the posterior border of the medial aspect of the lower limb, lateroposterior of the trunk and the posterior aspect of the axilla to the shoulder. It runs upward along the neck, to the retroauricular region and runs anterior to the forehead. It distributes at the temporal region and communicates with the Governor Vessel.

8.2 Function

The Yin Link Vessel links various Yin meridians. The Yang Link Vessel links various Yang meridians.

V. THE DIVERGENT MERIDIANS, COLLATERALS, MUSCLE REGIONS AND CUTANEOUS REGIONS

1. THE CONCEPT, RUNNING COURSE AND FUNCTION OF THE DIVERGENT MERIDIANS

1.1 Concept and running course

The twelve divergent meridians branch out from the twelve regular meridians. They are mainly distributed on the chest, abdomen and head. They derive from the regular meridians in the regions of four limbs that are above the elbow or knee, enter the thoracic and abdominal cavities, emerge to the body surface and ascend to the head and face. Then the Yin divergent meridians connect the internally–externally related Yang divergent meridians and join the six regular Yang meridians.

Each pair of internally–externally related divergent meridians forms a confluence. Altogether there are six confluences.

1.2 Functions

These are:

- to strengthen the relation of the two internally–externally related regular meridians inside the body

- to strengthen the relation between the body surface and the internal body, between the four limbs and the trunk

- to strengthen the relation between the twelve regular meridians, the head and face

- to broaden the indications of the twelve regular meridians

- to strengthen the relation of the three foot Yang meridians and three foot Yin meridians with the Heart.

2. THE CONCEPT AND FUNCTION OF COLLATERALS

2.1 Concept

The collaterals are branches from the twelve regular meridians and they are distributed on the body surface as a main component of all the collaterals. They play a leading role in the tiny collaterals of the body.

2.2 Functions

These are:

- to strengthen the relation of the two internally–externally related regular meridians

- to govern other collaterals and strengthen the relation between the anterior, posterior and lateral of the body

- to transport Qi and Blood so as to nourish the whole body.

3. THE CONCEPT AND FUNCTION OF THE MUSCLE REGIONS

3.1 Concept

They are the systems of the twelve regular meridians connecting the muscle and tendons.

3.2 Function

This is to control the bone and maintain the normal range of motion.

4. THE CONCEPT AND FUNCTION OF THE CUTANEOUS REGIONS

4.1 Concept

These are the areas of the skin distributed according to the running course of the meridians.

4.2 Function

Their function is to protect the body against external pathogens and reflect pathological changes.

CHAPTER

5

THE AETIOLOGY AND OCCURRENCE OF DISEASES

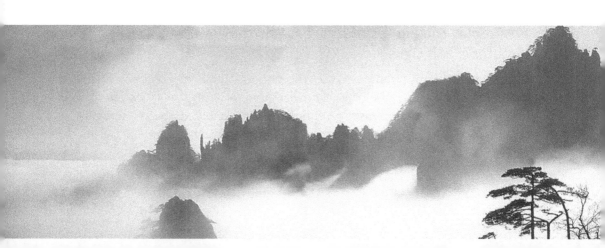

I. INTRODUCTION

Aetiology refers to the factors that disturb the relative balance of the body to cause diseases.

Occurrence of a disease is a process of struggle between the pathogenic factors that impair the body and the antipathogenic factors that protect the body.

II. AETIOLOGY

1. THE CONCEPT AND CLASSIFICATION OF AETIOLOGY

The pathogenic factors mainly include: six exogenous factors, epidemic factors, seven emotional factors, irregular food intake, overstrain and stress or lack of physical exercise, traumatic injuries, and insect or animal stings and bites, etc. These factors may cause diseases of a human body under certain conditions. Dr Zhang Zhongjing in the Han Dynasty wrote in his book, *Synopsis of Prescriptions of Golden Cabinet*:

> The causes of various diseases are divided into three types. Firstly, the pathogenic factors invade from the meridians and collaterals to the Zang Fu organs, which influence the internal body. Secondly, Blood circulation connects the four limbs and orifices of the body. Stagnation of these parts is because the skin is attacked. Thirdly, there are excessive sexual activity, incision, and insect or animal stings and bites.

Chen Wuze in the Song Dynasty put forward the Theory of Three Kinds of Aetiology, which held that the six exogenous factors belong to the *external cause*, emotional factors belong to the *internal cause*, and irregular food intake, overstrain and stress or lack of physical exercise, traumatic injuries and insect or animal stings and bites belong to *neither-internal-nor-external cause*.

1.1 Tracing the causes of a disease by differentiation of symptoms and signs

TCM holds that any syndrome is a reflection of a pathological body after it is influenced by a certain cause. The acknowledgment of TCM to aetiology is not only for the understanding of objective conditions that possibly work as factors causing diseases, but, more importantly, to provide a basis for treatment through tracing the causes of a disease by differentiation of symptoms and body signs from observation of clinical manifestations.

2. THE CONCEPT OF THE SIX EXOGENOUS FACTORS AND THEIR CHARACTERISTICS IN CAUSING DISEASES

The six exogenous factors include pathogenic Wind, Cold, Summer Heat, Damp, Dryness and Fire. Under normal conditions, Wind, Cold, Summer Heat, Damp, Dryness and Fire are called 'six types of Qi', namely six kinds of variation in the weather. When their effects is beyond the ability of the body to adapt, and they cause diseases, they are called the six exogenous factors. For example, the weather changes abnormally such as when it is too hot in summer or too cold in winter, or not hot in summer or not cold in winter. Or a type of Qi appears in the season when it should not dominate. To illustrate, in spring it should be warm, but instead it becomes cold. Or the weather changes too abruptly, such as it becoming abruptly cold or hot.

2.1 Common features of six exogenous factors in causing diseases

These are seasonal, combining, transforming and exogenous.

Seasonal: The six exogenous factors are related to seasons, climate or living places. For example, there is more pathogenic Wind in spring, more pathogenic Summer Heat in summer, more pathogenic Damp in late summer or early autumn, more pathogenic Dryness in late autumn, and more pathogenic Cold in winter. Besides, pathogenic Damp usually follows dwelling in a damp place. Pathogenic dry-Heat or Fire usually follows working in a place with a high temperature.

Combining: The six exogenous factors may affect the body individually or in combination of at least two of them. For example, there is a common cold due to pathogenic Wind Cold, diarrhoea due to pathogenic Damp Heat or Bi syndrome (painful joints) due to Wind, Cold and Damp.

Transforming: The six exogenous factors not only influence each other, but also transform into each other under certain conditions. Pathogenic Cold transmitting to the interior of the body may transform into Heat. Longstanding Summer Heat may transform into Dryness to consume Yin.

Exogenous: The six exogenous factors invade from the exterior via the skin, mouth and nose.

3. THE SIX EXOGENOUS FACTORS

3.1 Pathogenic Wind

3.1.1 Occurrence of pathogenic Wind

Wind is the predominant Qi of spring, but it may appear in all the four seasons. Therefore, although diseases due to pathogenic Wind occur the most frequently in spring, they also occur in other seasons. TCM holds that pathogenic Wind is a very important pathogenic factor in exogenous diseases. Pathogenic Wind usually invades from the exterior via the skin to cause external Wind syndrome.

3.1.2 Properties and pathological influences

Pathogenic Wind is a Yang pathogenic factor and is characterized by upward and outgoing dispersion and usually invades Yang parts of the body: Pathogenic Wind moves constantly with upward and outgoing dispersion, so it is regarded as a Yang pathogenic factor. It is all-pervasive during the invasion and causes the opening of pores over the body surface. It often attacks the upper portion of the body (head and face), Yang meridians and skin to open the pores. Clinical symptoms are headache, sweating and aversion to the wind, etc.

Pathogenic Wind occurs in gusts and is characterized by rapid change: Occurring in gusts means in diseases due to pathogenic Wind, the affected parts are migratory without fixed location. For example, in Bi syndrome due to pathogenic Wind, Cold and Damp, there is migratory pain of joints, which shows predominance of Wind and is called 'wandering Bi' or 'Wind Bi'. Rapid change means in diseases due to pathogenic Wind, the symptoms appear and disappear with abrupt onset. For example, in urticaria, there is itching of the skin in different parts of the body without fixed location. In exogenous diseases due to pathogenic Wind, there is abrupt onset of symptoms with rapid change. Thus, it was written in *Plain Questions* that pathogenic Wind occurs in gusts and is characterized by rapid change.

Pathogenic Wind is apt to associate itself with other pathogenic factors: Pathogenic Wind tends to associate itself with Cold, Damp, Dryness or Heat and form exogenous Wind Cold, Wind Heat or Wind Damp. It is thus a leading causative factor in exogenous diseases.

Property	Pathological influences	Clinical symptoms
A Yang pathogenic factor	Upward and outgoing dispersion, usually invading Yang parts of the body	Headache, sweating, aversion to Wind
Occurring in gusts, rapid change	Migratory, abrupt onset	Bi syndrome
Apt to associate itself with other pathogenic factors	Apt to associate with Cold, Damp, Dryness or Heat	Wind Cold Wind Heat Wind Damp

3.2 Pathogenic Cold

3.2.1 Occurrence and nature of pathogenic Cold

Cold is the predominant Qi of winter. The low winter temperature, wearing too little clothing when the temperature suddenly reduces, being caught in rain, and exposure to cold after sweating all provide chances for the development of pathogenic Cold. This is classified into external Cold and internal Cold.

External Cold refers to the invasion of exogenous pathogenic Cold and includes exogenous exterior syndrome and exogenous interior syndrome.

- Exogenous exterior syndrome means pathogenic Cold invades the skin and body surface, and obstructs the defensive Yang.

- Exogenous interior syndrome means pathogenic Cold directly invades the interior of the body, and impairs the Yang Qi of the Zang Fu organs.

Internal Cold is a pathological condition in which Yang Qi deficiency cannot warm the body.

External Cold and internal Cold influence each other. It is more likely for a body that is internally Cold due to Yang deficiency to be invaded by external Cold, while a longstanding external pathogenic Cold usually impairs Yang Qi to cause internal Cold.

3.2.2 Properties and pathological influences

Pathogenic Cold is a Yin pathogenic factor and is likely to consume Yang Qi: Pathogenic Cold is a manifestation caused by an excess of Yin. An excess of Yin leads to a Cold syndrome. Yang Qi usually restrains Yin, but when there is excessive Yin Cold, Yang Qi can not expel pathogenic Yin Cold. Instead, it is consumed by the Yin Cold, which is called 'excess of Yin affecting Yang'. So an invasion of pathogenic Cold is most likely to consume Yang Qi with Cold syndrome due to declining of Yang Qi. When external Cold invades the skin and body surface and obstructs the defensive Yang, the clinical manifestation is chills. When pathogenic Cold directly invades the Spleen and Stomach to impair Spleen Yang, the clinical manifestations are epigastric pain with a Cold sensation, vomiting and diarrhoea. When there is Yang deficiency of the Heart and Kidney with pathogenic Cold invading Shaoyang, clinical manifestations are chills, lying in a curled position, Cold limbs, diarrhoea with undigested food in the stool, clear urine in increased volume, and a feeble and thready pulse.

Pathogenic Cold is characterized by stagnation: The constant and free flow of Qi, Blood and Body Fluids in the body depends on the warming and promoting of Yang Qi. Excessive pathogenic Cold consumes Yang Qi to cause stagnation of Qi and Blood in the meridians due to the failure of warming and promoting. Pain occurs when there is stagnation. So a common symptom when pathogenic Cold invades the body is pain.

Pathogenic Cold is characterized by contraction: Contraction refers to constringency and contracture. When pathogenic Cold invades the body, it causes contraction of Qi, skin, meridians and collaterals, tendons and vessels. Invasion of pathogenic Cold to the skin and body surface causes closing of the pores so the defensive Yang cannot disperse, with manifestations of chills, fever and anhidrosis. Invasion of pathogenic Cold to the bood vessels causes stagnation of Qi and Blood, and contracture of bood vessels with manifestations of pain in the head and body and tense pulse. Invasion of pathogenic Cold to the meridians and collaterals and joints causes contracture in these parts, with manifestations of motor impairment or Cold in the extremities.

Pathogenic Cold

Property	Pathological influences	Clinical symptoms
A Yin pathogenic factor	Likely to consume Yang Qi	Chills, Cold limbs, thready pulse
Stagnation	Stagnation of Qi and Blood	Pain
Contraction	Constringency, contracture	Anhidrosis, lying in a curled position

3.3 Pathogenic Summer Heat
3.3.1 Concept

Summer Heat is the predominant Qi of summer and is transformed from Fire and Heat. It is especially seasonal and appears mainly from the Summer Solstice to the beginning of autumn. There is only external pathological Summer Heat and no internal Summer Heat.

3.3.2 Properties and pathological influences

Pathogenic Summer Heat is a Yang pathogenic factor with a hot property: Pathogenic Summer Heat is transformed from Fire and Heat in summer. Fire and Heat pertain to Yang, so pathological Summer Heat is a Yang pathogenic factor. Invasion of Summer Heat may cause a syndrome of Yang and Heat, with manifestations of high fever, irritability, red face or tongue, and surging pulse.

Pathogenic Summer Heat is characterized by upward direction and dispersion and consumes Qi and Body Fluid: Pathogenic Summer Heat is a Yang pathogenic factor, which features upward movement and dispersion. It usually invades the Qi directly to cause opening of the pores with polyhidrosis. Profuse sweating consumes Body Fluid with manifestations of thirst and a preference for drinks, yellow and scanty urine. Summer Heat also disturbs the Heart and Mind with manifestations of irritability and restlessness. There is an exhaustion of Qi together with Body Fluid during profuse sweating and thus causes Qi deficiency.

Pathogenic Summer Heat often combines with Damp: Rain and humidity often accompany the Heat of summer. So Summer Heat often combines with Damp to invade the body. Besides the Summer Heat syndrome of fever and thirst, there is also an accompanying syndrome due to retention of Damp with manifestations of lassitude, a suffocating feeling in the chest, nausea, and loose and hesitant stools.

Pathogenic Summer Heat

Property	Pathological influences	Clinical symptoms
Hot	A Yang pathogenic factor, excess Heat syndrome	High fever, thirst, red face and eyes, surging pulse
Upward direction and dispersion	Invading the head and eyes	Dizziness, blurred vision
	Disturbing the Heart and Mind	Heatstroke with sudden fainting and unconsciousness
	Opening of the pores	Polyhidrosis
Combining with Damp	Syndrome due to combination of Summer Heat and Damp	Fever indistinct at the first touch of the skin, thirst, general heaviness and lassitude, suffocating feeling in the chest, nausea, yellow and sticky coating

3.4 Pathogenic Damp

3.4.1 Concept

Damp is the predominant Qi of late summer – the period between summer and autumn. The hot weather steams the Water upwards to cause much Damp. Late summer is therefore the season in the year with the most Damp.

External Damp is due to the invasion of exogenous Damp in the human body.

Internal Damp is a pathological condition under which the dysfunction of the Spleen in transportation and transformation causes retention of water and Damp.

External Damp and internal Damp can influence each other. Invasion of external Damp may obstruct the Spleen to cause a dysfunction in transportation and transformation, which leads to the forming of internal Damp. On the other hand, if deficiency of Spleen Yang means that water and Damp cannot be transformed, it is more likely for external Damp to invade the body.

3.4.2 Properties and pathological influences

Pathogenic Damp is characterized by heaviness and turbidity: Damp is a substantial pathogenic factor that is weighty in nature. Its invasion of the body often gives rise to such symptoms as heaviness and a sensation of distention in the head, as if it was tightly bandaged. There is also heaviness of the body and four limbs. Due to invasion of pathogenic Damp to the skin, the clear Yang cannot ascend and there is disharmony between the nutrient and defensive systems. Due to the invasion of pathogenic Damp to the meridians and joints, Yang Qi cannot be distributed to these parts, with manifestations of numbness of the skin, arthralgia with fixed pain, which can be called 'fixed Bi' (in which Damp predominates). Turbidity is shown in the secretions. Invasion of pathogenic Damp often causes dirtiness in the face, loose stools, stools with pus and Blood, turbid urine or massive leucorrhoea.

Pathogenic Damp is a Yin pathogenic factor, which obstructs Qi circulation and impairs Yang: Pathological Damp is characterized by heaviness and turbidity, which are similar to the properties of Water, so it is a Yin pathogenic factor. Invasion of pathogenic Damp in the body stagnates the meridians and collaterals, and the Zang Fu organs and also obstructs Qi circulation, resulting in a disorder in the ascending and descending of Qi and stagnation of the meridians and collaterals. Clinical manifestations are fullness in the chest and epigastrium, scanty and hesitant urination, hesitant stool. Pathogenic Damp is a Yin pathogenic factor. Since a preponderance of Yin will consume Yang, an invasion of pathogenic Damp is most likely to impair Yang. As an important organ for transporting and transforming Water and Damp, the Spleen prefers Dryness to Damp. So exogenous pathogenic Damp usually obstructs the Spleen first, causing deficiency of the Spleen Yang in transportation and transformation, which results in retention of Water and Damp with manifestations of diarrhoea, scanty urine, oedema or ascites.

Pathogenic Damp is characterized by viscosity and stagnation: First, the syndrome due to pathogenic Damp is accompanied by viscous and sticky ejections or secretions. Second, diseases caused by pathogenic Damp are often lingering and longstanding, with long courses or recurrence.

Pathogenic Damp is characterized by downward direction and is likely to invade the Yin parts: Pathological Damp is characterized by downward direction. Diseases caused by pathogenic Damp are usually featured by symptoms in lower parts of the body such as oedema, which is more obvious in the lower extremities. Downward flow of pathogenic Damp may cause turbid stranguria, leucorrhoea, diarrhoea or dysentery.

Pathogenic Damp

Property	Pathological influences	Clinical symptoms
Heaviness and turbidity	Heaviness of the body	Heaviness of the head, trunk and four limbs, arthralgia with fixed pain
	Turbid secretions or ejections	Turbid urine, loose stool, stool with pus and Blood, dirtiness of the face
Viscosity and stagnation	Viscosity and stagnation of symptoms	Sticky and hesitant stool, hesitant urination, sticky secretions
	Long course of disease or recurrence	Fixed Bi, long course and recurrence of eczema
A Yin pathogenic factor	Obstructs Qi circulation, impairs Yang	Obstructs Qi circulation of the Spleen and Stomach with epigastric distention and anorexia, deficiency of Spleen Yang with diarrhoea and oedema
Downward direction	Invades lower parts of the body, symptoms in lower parts of the body	Turbid stranguria, leucorrhoea, diarrhoea, dysentery, oedema or ulceration of the lower extremities

3.5 Pathogenic Dryness
3.5.1 Concept

Dryness is the predominant Qi of autumn, a time when the weather becomes cool and dry with a lack of moisture in the air. Pathogenic Dryness usually invades the body via the mouth, nose or skin to further attack the Lungs or defensive system. It is classified into Warm Dryness and Cool Dryness. Some heat in summer remains in the early autumn, which combines with the Dryness to invade the human body, resulting in the syndrome of Warm Dryness. Some of the cold of winter appears in the late autumn, which combines with the Dryness to invade the human body, resulting in the syndrome of Cool Dryness.

3.5.2 Properties and pathological influences

The dry nature is apt to consume Body Fluid: With a dry property, invasion of external pathogenic Dryness is most likely to consume Body Fluid and cause insufficiency of Yin fluid. Clinical manifestations are thirst, dry throat, dry, rough and chapped skin, lustreless hair or body hair, scanty urine and dry stools.

Pathogenic Dryness is apt to impair the Lungs, which are delicate organs and prefers moisture to Dryness: The Lungs dominate Qi and control respiration in order to have a connection with the outside atmosphere. They also dominates the skin and body hair and open into the nose. So invasion of pathogenic Dryness via the mouth, nose or skin, and its consumption of Body Fluid, may impair the Lungs' dispersing and descending nature. Clinical manifestations are a dry cough with little sputum, sticky sputum that is difficult to expectorate, or Bloody sputum, whooping and chest pain.

Pathogenic Dryness

Property	Pathological influences	Clinical symptoms
Dry	Apt to consume Body Fluid	Dry mouth, lips, nose or throat, chapped skin, scanty urine, dry stools
	Apt to consume Lung Yin	Dry cough with little sputum, sticky sputum that is difficult to expectorate or Bloody sputum

3.6 Pathogenic Fire (Heat)

3.6.1 Concept

Pathogenic Fire, Heat and mild Heat are transformed from excessive Yang. They are of the same nature but different in intensity. Of these, Fire is the most severe, and mild Heat the least severe. Pathogenic Fire is classified into external and internal Fire.

External Fire is due to direct invasion of pathogenic Warmth and Heat.

Internal Fire may be transformed from excessive Yang Qi caused by disharmony of Qi, Blood, and Yin and Yang of the Zang Fu organs. Second, external pathogenic Wind, Cold, Summer Heat, Damp or Dryness, and emotional stimulation can also transform into Fire under certain conditions.

3.6.2 Properties and pathological influences

Pathogenic Fire (Heat) is a Yang pathogenic factor, which is characterized by upward movement: Yang is characterized by upward movement. Since pathogenic Fire always flares up, it has a Yang pathogenic factor. Clinical manifestations are high fever, aversion to heat, thirst, sweating, surging and rapid pulse. It also flares up to disturb mental activity, with manifestations of irritability, insomnia, mania, coma and delirium.

Pathogenic Fire (Heat) is apt to consume Qi and Body Fluid: Pathogenic Fire or Heat may drive Body Fluid outside the body and extract Yin fluid to cause consumption of Yin and Body Fluid. Clinical manifestations are thirst with a preference for drinking water, dry mouth or throat, yellow and scanty urine and dry stool, which is called 'excessive Fire impairing Qi'. Excessive Fire refers to Fire of an excess type transformed from hyperactivity of Yang Heat. It is apt to impair the antipathogenic Qi of the body and lead to a general declining of Qi and Body Fluid.

Pathogenic Fire (Heat) is apt to stir up Wind and disturb Blood: An invasion of pathogenic Fire or Heat may exhaust the Yin of the Liver and cause malnutrition of tendons and meridians, resulting in the internal disturbance of Liver Wind, known as 'extreme Heat stirring up Wind'. Clinical manifestations are high fever, coma, delirium, convulsions, upward gaze, stiffness of the neck, opisthotonos. Pathogenic Fire or Heat may cause extravasation by disturbing the Blood and therefore, haemorrhages may occur, such as haematemesis, epistaxis, haematochezia, haematuria and skin eruptions.

Pathogenic Fire (Heat) is apt to cause skin infections: Invasion of pathogenic Fire or Heat to the Blood layer may collect in the local area to cause infections such as carbuncles, furuncle, boils and ulcers. For example, ulcers with local redness, swelling, burning sensation and pain are caused by pathogenic Fire.

Pathogenic Fire

Property	Pathological influences	Clinical symptoms
Hot	A Yang pathogenic factor, excess Heat syndrome	High fever, red face, irritability, thirst, sweating, surging and rapid pulse
	Upward direction, mainly symptoms in the upper body	Fever, dizziness, headache, red face or eyes, sore throat, ulcers in the mouth or tongue
	Apt to consume Body Fluid and Qi	Thirst with preference for drinking Water, dry throat or lips, deep red tongue, lassitude, weakness
	Apt to stir up Wind	'Extreme Heat stirring up Wind' with high fever, convulsion, trismus, upward gaze, opisthotonos
	Apt to disturb Blood	'Heat causing extravasation of Blood,' haematemesis, epistaxis, haematuria, skin eruptions
	Apt to disturb the Heart and Mind	High fever, mania, coma, delirium
	Apt to cause skin infections	Carbuncles, furuncles, boils and ulcers with local redness, swelling, burning sensation and pain

4. PESTILENCE

4.1 Concept

Pestilence is a pathogenic factor with strong infectiousness.

4.2 Pathological influences

It is characterized by abrupt onset, severe and similar symptoms, and is extremely hot humid conditions, infectious and epidemic.

4.3 Related factors

These are:

- *Weather*: This refers to the abnormal change of the weather such as drought, humid fog and miasma, etc.

- *Environment and food*: This refers to polluted air, water, or food.

- Not immediately preventable and isolation is required.

5. THE SEVEN EMOTIONAL FACTORS

5.1 Concept

Mental activities related to emotions are classified in Traditional Chinese Medicine under: joy, anger, melancholy, worry, grief, fear and fright, which are known as the seven emotional factors.

Under normal conditions, the seven emotional factors will not cause disease. However, if the emotions are very sudden, intense or persistent, they are beyond the normal physiological accommodation of the body and cause disorder of Qi and Blood circulation, dysfunction of the Zang Fu organs and disorders of Yin and Yang, which lead to disease.

5.2 Relationship with the Qi and Blood of the Zang Fu organs

The emotional activities take the Qi and Blood of the Zang Fu organs as their material base, and they are also the outward manifestations in terms of mental activities that reflect the rise and fall of Qi and Blood as well as the functional activities of the Zang Fu organs. Different emotions have different influences on the Zang Fu organs and changes in Qi and Blood of the Zang Fu organs also influence emotions.

5.3 Pathological influences

These are as described below.

Internal organs are injured directly: Anger is related to the Liver, joy is related to the Heart, melancholy and grief are related to the Lungs, worry is related to the Spleen and fear and fright are related to the Kidneys. Emotions that are too intense and persistent can selectively injure different Zang Fu organs: anger injures the Liver, joy injures the Heart, melancholy and grief injure the Lungs, worry injures the Spleen, and fear and fright injure the Kidneys. However, the seven emotions are especially closely related to the Heart, which governs the mental activities. So the injury caused by the seven emotions to the Zang organs will first influence the Heart and Mind. The Liver's function in maintaining potency for the flow of Qi and storing Blood may regulate Qi and Blood and maintain a high mood. The Spleen and Stomach function as both a hinge for the ascending and descending of the Qi of the Zang Fu organs and the source for production of Qi and Blood. Clinically, disorders caused by the seven emotional activities are seen mainly in the Heart, Liver, and Spleen.

Qi circulation of Zang Fu organs is affected: Anger causes ascending of Qi. Excessive anger causes the Liver-Qi to ascend abnormally to the upper body, accompanied by Blood. Clinical manifestations are red face and eyes, haematemesis or even syncope and sudden fainting.

Joy causes slowing of Qi. This includes alleviating stress and causing laxation of Heart-Qi. Under normal circumstance, joy alleviates stress and circulates the nutrient and defensive layers that make people relaxed and happy. But excessive joy makes the Heart-Qi lax and the Mind cannot be housed. Clinical manifestations are lack of concentration or even mental confusion and mania.

Grief causes consumption of Qi. Excessive grief may consume the Lung-Qi and make people depressed.

Fear causes descending of Qi. Excessive fear may cause unconsolidation of the Kidney-Qi and descending of Qi. Clinical manifestations are incontinence of urine or stool, or flaccidity, and soreness of bones, and seminal emission if longstanding fear consumes the Essence.

Fright causes derangement of Qi. Sudden fright may impair the Heart to make the Mind lose its attachment. Clinical manifestations are anxiety and panic.

Worry causes stagnation of Qi. Excessive worry impairs the Spleen to cause stagnation. Worry germinates from the Spleen to the Heart, so excessive worry consumes the Heart and Mind and impairs the Spleen. Clinical manifestations are palpitations, poor memory, insomnia and dream-disturbed sleep due to malnutrition of the Heart and Mind. Besides, Qi stagnation causes the failure of the Spleen to transport and transform as well as dysfunctioning of the Stomach in receiving and digesting food, with manifestations of anorexia, epigastrium distention and loose stools.

Abnormal fluctuations of the emotions may worsen the state of a disease: A big fluctuation of emotions may worsen the states of a disease or exacerbate diseases very quickly. For example, when a person with a history of hypertension becomes angry about something, this causes sudden hyperactivity of the Liver Yang and an immediate increase of blood pressure, with manifestations of dizziness, sudden syncope, hemiplegia and deviation of the eyes and mouth. A fluctuation of emotions may also worsen the states of people suffering from Heart diseases.

6. IRREGULAR FOOD INTAKE, OVERSTRAIN AND STRESS, OR LACK OF PHYSICAL EXERCISE

6.1 Irregular food intake

Overeating or insufficient food intake: The amount of food intake should be appropriate. Both overeating or insufficient food intake can cause diseases.

Insufficient food intake doesn't provide enough nourishment. Lack of sources for production of Qi and Blood causes a syndrome of insufficient Qi and Blood. Moreover, it leads to weakness of the antipathogenic Qi, and other secondary syndromes may occur.

Overeating takes in more food than the Spleen and Stomach can digest and absorb and causes retention of food and epigastrium distention, belching of foul air, anorexia, vomiting and diarrhoea. Prolonged food retention may transform into Heat, which possibly obstructs Qi and Blood circulation, as well as the meridians, with manifestations of dysentery or haemorrhoids. Overeating of greasy and highly flavoured food is apt to transform into internal Heat leading to carbuncles, cellulitis or ulcers.

Intake of unclean food: Intake of unclean food causes various gastrointestinal diseases such as abdominal pain, vomiting, diarrhoea, or dysentery. Or it may cause parasitic diseases, such as ascariasis, or oxyuriasis with manifestations of abdominal pain, a preference for eating strange food, sallow complexion and emaciation.

Indulgence in particular food: First this refers to eating food that is too Cold or too hot. Eating Cold or uncooked food injures the Yang of the Spleen and Stomach, leading to internal Cold and Damp with manifestations of abdominal pain or diarrhoea; eating pungent, warm, dry and hot food leads to retention of Heat in the gastrointestine with manifestations of thirst, distending pain in the abdomen, constipation, or haemorrhoids.

Second, it refers to overindulgence in some of the five flavours of food. There should be proper selection of the five flavours of food during daily diet and especially during the course of diseases. Indulgence in one flavour over a long period leads to hyperfunction of the corresponding Zang organ and gradually injures the internal organs and cause disease.

6.2 Overstrain and stress or lack of physical exercise

Proper work and exercise are good for the circulation of Qi and Blood and strengthening of the body constitution. Necessary rest can remove tiredness and restore physical and mental strength. Overstrain and stress, or lack of physical exercise can also cause diseases.

6.2.1 Overstrain and stress

Overstrain and stress includes physical strain, mental stress and excessive sexual activity.

Physical strain: This refers to the overuse of physical strength over a long period, which consumes Qi with manifestations of whooping, short breath, sweating, lassitude and emaciation.

Mental stress: This refers to worry that consumes and injures the Heart and Spleen. Blood is the material base of mental activities. The Heart dominates Blood and houses the Mind. Worry bothers the Mind so that is consumes the Heart Blood and injures the Spleen-Qi. Malnutrition of the Heart and Mind causes palpitations, poor memory, insomnia or dream-disturbed sleep. Deficiency of the Spleen in transporting and transforming causes abdominal distention, anorexia or loose stools.

Excessive sexual activity: The Kidneys store Essence, which should not be overly tired. Too frequent sexual activity will consume Kidney Essence, with manifestations of soreness and weakness of the lumbar region and knees, dizziness, tinnitus, lassitude and listlessness, seminal emission, premature ejaculation or impotence.

6.2.2 Lack of physical exercise

People need to do appropriate exercise every day in order to maintain the smooth circulation of Qi and Blood. Lack of physical exercise for a long time causes poor appetite, general weakness, lassitude, obesity, or palpitations, shortness of breath and sweating after exertion, and other secondary diseases.

7. TRAUMATIC INJURIES

7.1 Concept

Traumatic injuries include: gunshot injuries, incisions, contusions, sprains, scalds and burns, frostbite, and insect or animal stings and bites.

7.2 Pathological influences

Incisions, contusions and sprains: In mild cases, these cause Blood stasis, swelling and pain of the skin and muscles, haemorrhage, bone fracture or dislocation. In severe cases, they injure the internal organs or the head, and cause general symptoms, due to the loss of too much Blood, such as unconsciousness, convulsions and collapse of Yang.

Scalds and burns: These are caused by Heat, boiling Water, or hot liquids. In mild cases, the skin is injured, with redness, swelling, hotness, and pain. Or the skin is dry, or there is blistering and severe pain of the skin. In severe cases, the muscle, tendon and bone are injured, with analgesia. The surface of the wound looks like leather with a white colour similar to wax, a brown colour, or a colour similar to carbonization. In the most severe cases, the surface of the wound is extremely large. As well as local symptoms (because of the severe pain, internal attacking of toxic Fire and evaporation, and effusion of Body Fluid) there is also irritability, fever, dry mouth, thirst, scanty urine or even death.

Frostbite: This refers to the general or local injury of the body resulting from exposure to freezing or subfreezing temperatures. Initially, the local skin is pale, Cold and numb because a Cold dominating contraction causes contracture of the meridians and collaterals and stagnation of Qi and Blood, which cannot warm and nourish the skin. Then there is swelling and a purple colour, extreme itching with a burning sensation, or blisters of various sizes, which infect easily after they break.

Insect or animal stings and bites: These are from poisonous snakes, fierce beasts, dogs, scorpions, or bees. In mild cases, there is redness, swelling, pain and bleeding of the local skin. In severe cases, the internal organs are injured or death even occurs due to excessive haemorrhage.

8. STAGNATION OF PHLEGM OR BLOOD

Stagnation of Phlegm or Blood is a pathological product formed during the course of diseases after a certain pathogenic factor invades the body. This acts on the body directly or indirectly to cause many symptoms and are also included into pathogenic factors.

8.1 Stagnation of Phlegm

8.1.1 Concept

Phlegm (Tan Yin) is a pathological product that is retained inside the body as a result of a disturbance of the water metabolism. The thick and turbid is called 'Tan', while the thin and clear is called 'Yin'.

8.1.2 Classification

Classification of tan:

- *Visible Tan* refers to the sputum people cough or vomit out

- *Invisible Tan* stagnates in the Zang Fu organs, meridians and collaterals and certain local areas, and can be diagnosed through observation of the clinical syndrome or treatment.

Classification of Yin: See the table below.

Classification of Yin

Location	Symptoms
In the chest and hypochondrium	Fullness in the chest and hypochondrium, dull pain during cough, fullness in the affected intercostal space
In the chest and diaphragm	Stuffiness in the chest, palpitation, can't lie in a horizontal position
In the skin	Oedema of skin, anhidrosis, pain of body
In the gastrointestine	Fullness in the epigastrium, borborygmus, vomiting of clear sputum

8.1.3 Formation

Retention of Body Fluid is induced either from a disturbed function of the water metabolism, or a disturbed vaporizing function of Qi, which is often due to a dysfunction of the Zang Fu organs especially the Lungs, Spleen, Kidneys or Triple Burner. The causative factors might be the six exogenous pathogenic factors, indulgent food intake, or the seven emotional factors.

Most Zang Fu organs, especially the Lungs, Spleen, Kidneys and Triple Burner, are closely related to water metabolism.

As we know, the Lungs dominate dispersing, and descending of Qi, and regulate the water passages, which distributes Body Fluid to the whole body, whilst the Spleen is mainly responsible for transportation of Body Fluid, Kidney Yang is responsible for vaporizing, and the Triple Burner is the passage for water metabolism. Any of those organs can lose its normal function, such as the Lungs losing their function of dispersing and descending, the Spleen losing its function of transportation, the Kidneys losing their function of controlling urination and separating the clear from the turbid, and the Triple Burner losing its ability to regulate the water passages. Each of these cases can lead to retention of Body Fluid or the production of Damp in the interior of the body.

8.1.4 Characteristic of causative factors

Characteristics for Phlegm-induced syndromes:

Characteristics	Main manifestations and signs	
Blocking Qi and Blood circulation	Obstruction of Phlegm in Lungs	Stuffiness in chest, cough, asthma
	Retention of Damp in Middle Burner	Distention in epigastrium, nausea and vomiting
	Phlegm obstructs meridians and collaterals	Numbness and limited functions of four limbs
	Local obstruction	Subcutaneous nodules, scrofula, cellulites, multiple abscesses
Resulting in large variety of diseases, often manifested as dramatic changes	Many diseases are related to Phlegm, especially those rarely encountered diseases	
Prolonged continuation of disease	Cough, asthma, dizziness and vertigo, scrofula, chest Bi, epilepsy, multiple abscess, hemiplegia, subcutaneous nodules, cellulites	
Easily disturbed Mind	Mental disorders such as mental depression or dullness, insomnia, easily getting angry, weeping and laughing without an apparent reason, or mania in severe cases	
More likely with rolling pulse and sticky tongue-coating		

Characteristics for fluid-induced syndromes: When fluid accumulates in the intestines there will be symptoms like borborygmus; if it attacks the chest and hypochondrium there can be distention in the chest or chest pain induced by cough or asthma; when it obstructs the diaphragm, there are symptoms such as stuffiness in the chest, the patient being unable to lie down on the bed due to severe cough, and general swelling may occur. In cases where pathogenic fluid floods to the skin and body surface then oedema, anhidrosis, and a sensation of heaviness and pain may present in the body.

8.2 Blood stasis
8.2.1 Concept
Blood stasis refers to retention of Blood inside the body, including Blood accumulating outside bood vessels, or accumulation of Blood in the meridians or Zang Fu organs.

8.2.2 Formation

Blood stasis can be caused either by Qi deficiency or stagnation of Qi, or by Cold or Heat in the Blood: Qi is the commander of the Blood and deficiency or stagnation of Qi implies weakness of Qi in propelling Blood normally. Also, invasion of pathogenic Cold into the bood vessels, or the invasion of pathogenic Heat to the Ying (nutrient) stage may lead to contraction, or to the strife of Heat with Blood, resulting in stagnation of the Blood.

Blood stasis can also be induced by traumatic injury or internal injury, Qi deficiency or Heat in the Blood disturbing the normal circulation of Blood: when the Blood circulates outside its normal passage or accumulates inside the body then Blood stasis can occur (see Figure 5.1).

8.2.3 Pathogenic features

Pain: Often localized stabbing pain, which is worse at night.

Mass: Black and blue at local region, in chronic conditions an accumulation of stagnant Blood in the local area forms a tumourous mass, which has a fixed position and is firm on palpation.

Bleeding: The colour of flow is purplish dark, and may exhibit clots.

Pulse: The pulse is thready, hesitant, deep and wiry or knotted.

Inspection: Dark complexion, dry skin, purplish lips and nails; to some extent symptoms like ecchymosis or petechiae, or varicose veins below the tongue may present.

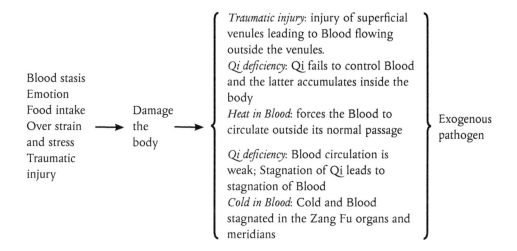

Figure 5.1

Manifestations of Blood stasis in different areas

Area of Accumulation	Symptoms and signs
Accumulated in Heart	Palpitation, stuffiness in chest, cardiac pain, purplish lips and nails
Accumulated in Lungs	Chest pain, cough with Blood
Accumulated in Stomach and intestine	Blood vomited out is the colour of coffee, and the stool is dark-coloured
Accumulated in Liver	Fullness sensation and pain in hypochondrium
Stagnant Blood attacks the Heart	Mania
Accumulated in uterus	Pain in lower abdomen, irregular menstruation, amenorrhea, purplish dark flow, may exhibit clots, sometime uterine bleeding may present
Accumulated in four limbs and terminals	Dislocation of joints, gangrene
Accumulated in skin and hair	Local swelling and pain with cyanosis

III. PRINCIPLES FOR THE ONSET OF DISEASES

1. BASIC PRINCIPLES FOR THE ONSET OF DISEASES

When the functions of the Zang Fu organs, meridians and collaterals are normal, the Qi and Blood, Yin and Yang are in proper balance, and the human body remains healthy – that is to say diseases will not occur unless the body is invaded by pathogenic factors. Invasion of pathogenic Qi results in conflict between the antipathogenic Qi and the pathogenic Qi, which destroys the Yin–Yang harmony of the body and causes functional disturbance of the Zang Fu organs and meridians, and derangement of Qi and Blood.

1.1 Pathogenic Qi, antipathogenic Qi and the onset of diseases

'Antipathogenic Qi' refers to the functional activities of the human body (such as the functions of the Zang Fu organs, the meridians and collaterals, and the Qi and the Blood), its ability to resist disease and its ability for rehabilitation.

'Pathogenic Qi' refers to various causative factors leading to the onset of disease.

The onset and progression of disease can be generalized as being due to conflict between Xie (pathogenic) Qi and Zheng (antipathogenic) Qi.

1.1.1 Antipathogenic Qi is primary, being the internal factor that allows the invasion of the external factor

Plain Questions states: 'Pathogenic Qi cannot invade the body if the antipathogenic Qi remains strong.' Another paragraph in the same book comments 'Antipathogenic Qi must be weak if invasion of pathogenic Qi takes place.'

1.1.2 Pathogenic Qi also plays an important role as a condition for the onset of diseases

Traditional Chinese Medicine not only pays great attention to the role of antipathogenic Qi during the onset of the disease but also realizes the importance of pathogenic Qi, which means the latter may also play a leading role in certain conditions. For instance, invasion can be caused by high temperature and voltage from electrical current, chemical poison, gunshots, frostbite, and insect or animal bites, as well as epidemic factors. In these conditions, although antipathogenic Qi is strong, disease can still occur.

1.1.3 The result of conflict determines whether there will be disease or not

Disease will not occur when antipathogenic Qi wins the battle.

When antipathogenic Qi is strong enough to resist the invasion of pathogenic Qi, or antipathogenic Qi can eliminate the invaded pathogenic Qi, then disease will not occur.

Disease will occur when pathogenic Qi wins the battle. When pathogenic Qi exceeds antipathogenic Qi, it will result in dysfunction of the Zang Fu organs, disharmony of Yin and Yang, and derangement of Qi and Blood, thus leading to the onset of disease.

The relationship between disease and antipathogenic Qi: Syndromes of an excess type are likely to occur if there is both hyperactivity of pathogenic Qi and an sufficiency of antipathogenic Qi. syndromes of deficiency type, or syndromes of deficiency mixed with excess, are likely to occur if there is an excess of pathogenic Qi and a deficiency of antipathogenic Qi.

The relationship between disease and the nature of pathogenic Qi: Generally speaking, an invasion of pathogenic Yang Qi can consume Yin in the body, thus resulting in an excess syndrome; and an invasion of pathogenic Yin Qi can injure Yang in the body, thus resulting in an excess syndrome of Cold type or syndrome of Cold and Damp.

The relationship between disease and severity of pathogenic Qi: In the onset of diseases pathogenic Qi is an important factor which determines the severity of the disease alongside the general condition of the constitution of the body – that is, the weaker the pathogenic Qi, the milder the disease will be, and vice versa.

The relationship between disease and an affected area: Disease will vary if the invaded area is different. Some diseases may affect tendons, bones or vessels; others may invade the Zang Fu organs.

2. THE ENVIRONMENT AND THE ONSET OF DISEASES

'Outer environment' refers to the living and working environment, including climate change, geographic features, sanitation, etc.

Inner environment refers to body resistance.

2.1 Outer environment and the onset of disease

2.1.1 Climate

Diseases caused by the six exogenous pathogenic Qi or epidemic Qi are related to climate changes. The spring is often Windy, the summer is Hot, the late summer is accompanied by Damp Heat, the autumn is often Dry and the winter is characterized by Cold. The onset of epidemic diseases is closely related to seasonal changes in the weather, especially when there are abnormal climate changes – in other words, epidemic diseases only take place if the climatic changes are either extreme or sudden. For instance, epidemic parotitis (mumps), and whooping cough, are more often seen in winter or spring.

2.1.2 Geographic factors

Geographic and natural conditions determine the category of commonly encountered or frequently encountered diseases in a particular area.

2.1.3 Living and working environment

Living conditions, the quality of water, air and noise are all related to the onset of diseases.

2.1.4 Others

These include traumatic injury, insect or animal bites, mental stimulation, etc.

2.2 Inner environment and the onset of disease

Pathogenic factors are the main conditions for the onset of disease, while insufficiency of antipathogenic Qi is the primary cause of the disease. Generally speaking, body constitution and vitality determine the strength of antipathogenic Qi.

2.2.1 The relationship between body constitution and antipathogenic Qi

A strong constitution refers to the vital activity of the Zang Fu organs, including Essence, Qi, Blood, Body Fluids, and antipathogenic Qi to be sufficient.

One's constitution is closely related to one's congenital foundation, one's food intake and the amount of physical exercise one takes. If the body constitution is strong enough, the functional activity of the Zang Fu organs including Essence, Qi, Blood and Body Fluids are sufficient, and so the antipathogenic Qi will be vital too. If the body constitution is weak, the function of the Zang Fu organs will decline, thus antipathogenic Qi will be weakened. Therefore strengthening body resistance is beneficial in preventing the onset of disease.

2.2.2 The relationship between vital energy and antipathogenic Qi

One's vital activity can be influenced by emotional factors. If one is in a good mood, the circulation of Qi retains its smooth flow, and Qi and Blood and the Zang Fu organs are coordinating and functioning well, and so the antipathogenic Qi is vital. If on the other hand, one is emotionally depressed, the Qi circulation is obstructed, there is imbalanced Yin and Yang and deranged Qi and Blood, which will lead to dysfunction of the Zang Fu organs, thus leading to declined vitality of antipathogenic Qi. Regulating one's emotions may therefore strengthen antipathogenic Qi, and further prevent the onset of diseases.

PATHOGENESIS

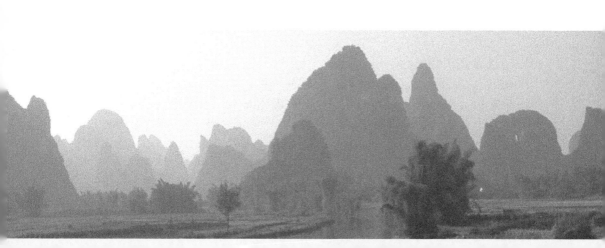

I. THE PROSPERITY AND DECLINE OF PATHOGENIC QI AND ANTIPATHOGENIC QI

The study of pathogenesis concerns the actual bodily processes whereby disease occurs, develops and changes.

1. THE PROSPERITY AND DECLINE OF PATHOGENIC QI AND ANTIPATHOGENIC QI

The strength of pathogenic Qi and antipathogenic Qi in the process of disease determines whether a syndrome is of a deficiency type or of an excess type.

1.1 The strength and equilibrium between the external environment and the human body is not static, but is in a state of constant self-adjustment

Generally speaking, if external influences exceed the powers of adaptability of the organism, then equilibrium will be lost. Furthermore, if the physiological activity of the human body remains normal, disease will not occur. The interconsuming of pathogenic Qi and antipathogenic Qi will determine whether a disease is of an excess type or a deficiency type; according to *Plain Questions*: 'Hyperactivity of the pathogenic factor causes excess; consumption of essential Qi causes deficiency.'

1.1.1 Excess

Excess refers to hyperactivity of the pathogenic factor, and therefore syndromes of excess type refer to pathological conditions in which the pathogenic factor is hyperactive, while the antipathogenic Qi remains strong. This is commonly seen in the early and middle stages of diseases that are due to invasion of the exogenous pathogenic factors, and diseases caused by retention of Phlegm fluid, stagnant Blood, and Water Damp, as well as retention of food. Symptoms and signs are high fever, mania, sonorous voice, coarse breathing, distention and fullness in the chest and abdomen, pain aggravated by pressure, constipation or dysuria, and pulse of excess type.

1.1.2 Deficiency

Deficiency mainly refers to insufficiency of antipathogenic Qi, which is the pathological reaction dominated by the decline of antipathogenic Qi. This is commonly seen in diseases resulting from prolonged weakness of body constitution, poor function of the Zang Fu organs, and deficiency of Qi, Blood and Body Fluids due to a lingering disease. Symptoms and signs are listlessness, pallor, palpitations, shortness of breath, a feverish sensation in the Five Centres, or aversion to cold, cold limbs, spontaneous sweating, night sweating, pain alleviated by pressure, and pulse of deficiency type.

1.1.3 Complications of deficiency and excess

When deficiency of the antipathogenic Qi and excess of the pathogenic Qi manifest at the same time, this is known as a syndrome complicated with deficiency and excess. Although the pathogenic factor in syndromes of an excess type may gradually subside, the antipathogenic Qi is already injured due to delayed or incorrect treatment, thus transforming syndromes of excess type into syndromes of deficiency type, or from deficiency to excess in other circumstances. False phenomena may appear in syndromes of deficiency type and those of excess type. True excess with false deficiency refers to a syndrome of excess type that is accompanied by symptoms and signs similar to a syndrome of deficiency type, which is often due to obstruction in meridians and collaterals, thus the Qi and Blood cannot disperse outward. True deficiency with false excess refers to a syndrome of deficiency type that is accompanied by symptoms and signs similar to a syndrome of excess type. It is often due to poor function of the Zang Fu organs, and insufficiency of Qi and Blood in transformation and transportation.

2. THE TRANSFORMATION OF THE DISEASE

The struggle between pathogenic Qi and antipathogenic Qi determines the onset, progression and transformation of the disease. If antipathogenic Qi wins the battle then the disease will get better or can be cured; if pathogenic Qi wins the battle then the disease will get worse or the patient may die. In some cases the strength of pathogenic Qi and antipathogenic Qi is comparatively equal and therefore the disease may change from acute to chronic, becoming a prolonged illness.

II. DISHARMONY OF YIN-YANG

1. CONCEPT

The normal interconsuming–supporting relationship is disturbed by either a preponderance or disturbance of Yin and Yang. Disharmony of Yin and Yang refers to pathological changes involving either excess or deficiency of Yin or Yang, which occur when the body is invaded by pathogenic Qi. Disease will not occur unless the body is invaded by pathogenic factors which cause derangement of Yin and Yang in the interior. As all the Zang Fu organs, meridians, Qi and Blood are classified in terms of Yin and Yang; exterior and interior, ascending and descending of Qi reflect Yin and Yang contradictions, and thus Yin and Yang form a pair of principles used to generalize categories of syndromes. All the contradictions and changes occurring in the disease process can be generalized in terms of Yin and Yang.

2. EXCESS OF YIN-YANG

Hyperactivity of pathogenic Qi causes syndromes of an excess type. Excess of Yang occurs if there is excess of exogenous pathogenic Yang Qi, while if there is an excess of exogenous pathogenic Yin then excess of Yin occurs. The clinical manifestations show that 'Excessive Yang produces Heat, while excessive Yin leads to Cold.'

2.1 Yang in excess

Yang in excess refers to the pathological condition of the human body that is characterized by signs of excessive Yang, hyperfunction of the Zang Fu organs, and excessive Heat in the body.

Aetiology: It is mainly manifested as excessive Heat syndrome that is Yang in excess while Yin is still not deficient. When Yang pathogenic factors cause disease this will give rise to Heat syndrome, thus symptoms such as high fever, redness of face and eyes may be seen. If there is excessive Yang, whilst Yin is relatively insufficient, then the disease is excess Heat syndrome; if Yin fluid is consumed while Yang is in excess, Yin turns from relative insufficiency to deficiency, therefore the disease changes from excess Heat syndrome to deficient Heat syndrome, or excess Heat combined with Yin deficiency.

2.2 Yin in excess

Yin in excess refers to the pathological condition of the human body characterized by hyperactivity of Yin, hypofunction of internal organs, and insufficiency of Heat. There are symptoms showing Yin and Cold syndromes.

Aetiology: It is mainly manifested as excessive Cold syndrome that is Yin in excess while Yang is still not deficient. When Yin pathogenic factors cause disease, this will give rise to Cold syndrome; thus symptoms such as aversion to Cold, Cold limbs, and pale tongue may be seen. If there is excessive Yin and deficiency of Yang, then the symptoms mainly show insufficiency of Yang Qi.

3. DEFICIENCY OF YIN-YANG

'Exhaustion of vital Essence brings on deficiency syndromes.' Deficiency syndrome refers to consumption of Essence, Qi, Blood and Body Fluids, or hypofunctions of human activity, and dysfunction of the Zang Fu organs, as well as dysfunctions of the meridians and collaterals. 'Deficiency of Yang causes excessive Yin, leading to Cold syndrome, while deficiency of Yin causes hyperactivity of Yang, leading to Heat syndrome.'

3.1 Deficiency of Yin

Deficiency of Yin refers to insufficiency of Essence, Blood and Body Fluid. The human body is in hyperfunction but of a deficiency type, as the relative hyperfunctioning of Yang is because Yin fails in controlling Yang.

Aetiology: Yin deficiency reduces its functions of moisturizing and calming down. When Yin fails to control Yang this will lead to Heat syndrome of a deficiency type. Yin deficiency is mainly manifested as deficiency of Liver and Kidney Yin, as Kidney Yin is considered essential for Yin in the body and so plays an important role in deficiency syndrome of Yin. As Yin cannot control Yang, there will be pathological manifestations showing internal Heat or Fire due to Yin deficiency, or hyperactivity of Yang. Symptoms and signs are feverish sensations in the Five Centres, flushed cheeks, night sweating, dry throat, red tongue with scanty coating, and thready, rapid and weak pulse.

Comparison of Yin deficiency and hyperactivity of Yang

	Deficiency and excess	Aetiology	Progression of the disease
Heat induced by Yin deficiency	Deficiency with Heat, but dominated by deficiency	No distinct reason showing attack by Heat	Slow onset and progress gradually
Heat induced by hyperactivity of Yang	Mainly manifested with Heat, no distinct evidence showing deficiency	With evidence showing Heat attack	Abrupt onset and progresses rapidly

3.2 Deficiency of Yang

Deficiency of Yang refers to consumption of Yang Qi, which body function and metabolism reduced. There are signs showing insufficiency of Heat.

Aetiology: Deficiency of Yang leads to relative excess of Yin. When Yang fails to control Yin it will lead to deficiency and Cold syndrome. In the case of Yang deficiency, deficiency of Spleen and Kidney Yang is more common. Kidney Yang is the fundamental Yang in the whole body, and therefore deficiency of Kidney Yang is inevitable when there is hypofunction of Yang. When Yang fails to control Yin, the warming function of Yang is reduced, leading to reduced function of the Zang Fu organs, and retention of Blood and Body Fluids, thus producing internal Cold, which is of a deficiency type. Symptoms such as pale complexion, aversion to cold, cold limbs, pale tongue, and slow pulse may present; meanwhile symptoms showing deficiency will also present, such as patients preferring to lie down, profuse urine and diarrhoea.

Comparison of Yang deficiency and hyperactivity of Yin

	Deficiency and excess	Aetiology	Progression of the disease
Cold induced by Yang deficiency	Deficiency with Cold, mainly dominated by deficiency	No distinct sign showing Cold attack	Slow onset and progresses gradually
Cold induced by hyperactivity of Yin	Mainly Cold, no distinct sign showing deficiency	With Cold attack	Abrupt onset and progresses rapidly

4. MUTUAL CONSUMPTION OF YIN AND YANG

Mutual consumption of Yin and Yang refers to consumption of Yin or Yang that affects the opposite side, leading to insufficiency of both Yin and Yang.

4.1 Yin consuming Yang

Yin consuming Yang refers to insufficiency of Yin fluid leading to malnutrition of Yang Qi – thus Yin and Yang are both deficient, but the condition is dominated by Yin deficiency.

4.2 Yang consuming Yin

Yang consuming Yin refers to insufficiency of Yang Qi leading to malnutrition of Yin – thus Yin and Yang are both deficient, but the condition is mainly characterized by Yang deficiency.

5. YIN OR YANG KEPT EXTERNALLY

For various reasons either Yin or Yang goes to its extreme, which keeps the opposite part outside. Qi in Yin and Yang fails to be maintained, which results in true Cold with pseudo-Heat or true Heat with pseudo-Cold.

5.1 Extreme Yin keeps Yang externally

Extreme Yin keeping Yang externally refers to the pathological condition of extreme Yin expelling Yang to float outside, in which the Qi in Yin and Yang fails to be maintained, resulting in true Cold with pseudo-Heat. The root cause of the disease is extreme Yin in the interior expelling Yang outside, thus this is often manifested as flushed cheeks, polylogia, irritability, thirst, and a full pulse without root.

5.2 Extreme Yang keeps Yin externally

Extreme Yang keeping Yin externally refers to the pathological condition of extreme Yang expelling Yin outside. Yang Qi may then not reach the four limbs, resulting in true Heat with pseudo-Cold, and thus symptoms such as cold limbs and deep pulse may present.

6. COLLAPSE OF YIN AND COLLAPSE OF YANG

Collapse of Yin refers to pathological conditions resulting from a massive consumption of Yin fluid. Collapse of Yang refers to pathological conditions caused by extreme exhaustion of Yang Qi in the body. Both collapse of Yin and collapse of Yang are critical syndromes in the process of a disease.

6.1 Collapse of Yang

Collapse of Yang refers to pathological conditions caused by extreme exhaustion of Yang Qi in the body, which is a critical syndrome in the process of a disease. Symptoms indicating extreme Cold and deficiency may present, such as cold and profuse sweating, pale complexion, listlessness, cold limbs, an aversion to cold, feeble breath, and fading pulse.

6.2 Collapse of Yin

Collapse of Yin refers to pathological conditions caused by extreme exhaustion of Yin fluid in the body, which is a critical syndrome in the process of a disease. Symptoms such as irritability, asthma, thirst, great loss of sweat, warm hands and feet, and rapid pulse may be seen.

As Yin and Yang depend upon each other, in the case of collapse of Yin, the Yang Qi has nothing to depend upon, therefore it dissipates from the body. In collapse of Yang, Yin fluid is also consumed. Collapse of Yin may lead to the rapid collapse of Yang, and vice versa. In either case, the patient will die due to the dissociation of Yin and Yang.

III. DYSFUNCTION OF QI AND BLOOD

Dysfunction of Qi and Blood refers to the abnormal function of Qi in its movement and activity, caused by consumption of Qi or Blood.

1. DEFICIENCY OF QI

Deficiency of Qi refers to the pathological condition caused by exhaustion of Qi or failure in Qi production so that antipathogenic Qi is weakened, and functioning of the Zang Fu organs declines.

Formation:

- Congenital deficiency, or malnutrition of acquired foundation.
- Dysfunction of Lungs, Spleen and Kidneys leading to failure in Qi production.
- Prolonged illness, or overstrain and stress.

Characteristic: Qi is too weak to defend against the invasion of pathogenic factors. Its checking function and Qi activity is impaired.

Clinical manifestations:

- In case of weakness of defensive Qi, it fails to control the opening and closing of pores, thus the patient may suffer from chills, spontaneous sweating, and more easily catch Cold.
- Deficiency of Spleen-Qi in transformation and transportation results in poor appetite, diarrhoea, lassitude, malnutrition of the four limbs, and general fatigue.
- Deficiency of Heart-Qi also implies weakness of Qi in propelling Blood normally. Hence palpitations, and weak pulse may present.
- If Lung-Qi is weak and thus fails in its function of respiration, shortness of breath and asthma may occur.
- Kidney-Qi deficiency may result in failure of Qi to be taken into the body. Symptoms such as inhaling more than exhaling, seminal emission and enuresis may present.

When Qi fails to promote circulation there will be symptoms such as retention of Damp or Body Fluid, and stagnation of Blood presenting in the body.

2. DISTURBED QI ACTIVITY

Disturbed Qi activity refers to pathological changes in coordination and balance due to the dysfunction of Qi in ascending and descending.

2.1 Stagnation of Qi

Stagnation of Qi refers to the pathological state of a certain Zang Fu organ, or of meridians and collaterals when as a result Qi is retarded and obstructed.

Formation:

- Emotional depression.

- Substantial obstruction caused by Phlegm, Damp, food and Blood stagnation.

- Invasion of exogenous pathogenic factors, which obstructs the Qi circulation; or dysfunction of the Zang Fu organs leading to stagnation of Qi.

- Qi is too weak to circulate normally, leading to stagnation of Qi.

Regulating Qi activity depends on the ascending of Liver and Spleen-Qi, and the descending of Lung and Stomach-Qi. When Qi stagnates in the Zang Fu organs, there will be stagnation of Lung-Qi, Liver-Qi or stagnation of Spleen and Stomach-Qi.

2.2 Perversion of Qi

An upward attack of Qi refers to the pathological state caused by disturbed Qi activity in ascending and descending, which results in upward attacking of Qi from the Zang Fu organs.

Formation: This is often induced from emotional injury, improper food intake, invasion of exogenous pathogenic factors or retention of turbid Phlegm.

Clinical manifestations: This mainly affects the Zang Fu organs, particularly the Lungs, Stomach and Liver.

- Perversion of Lung-Qi may impair the normal function of Lung-Qi in descending, thus leading to hiccups and asthma.

- Perversion of Stomach-Qi may disturb the function of Stomach-Qi in descending, thus resulting in nausea, vomiting, hiccups and belching.

- Perversion of Liver-Qi may result in the dysfunction of Liver-Qi in flowing smoothly, and there will be distention and redness of head and face, and the patient may become angry easily. In severe cases, symptoms such as coughing with Blood, vomiting with Blood and coma may present.

2.3 Sinking of Qi

This is one kind of Qi deficiency, manifested as failure in ascending Qi.

Formation: Congenital deficiency, or prolonged illness may consume Qi in the body, leading to Spleen-Qi deficiency. Therefore the clear Yang fails to ascend.

Clinical manifestations: Deficiency of Qi is manifested as lassitude, shortness of breath, pallor and weak pulse.

Failure of clear Yang in ascending leads to malnutrition to the head and eyes, resulting in dizziness, blurred vision and tinnitus.

If Qi cannot ascend, there are symptoms such as gastroptosis and renal ptosis, and prolapse of the uterus or anus.

Manifestations showing that clear Yang failing to ascend and turbid Qi is failing to descend can be distention and a bearing down sensation of lower abdomen, tenesmus, etc.

2.4 Qi block or collapse

This is the pathological state showing an abnormal condition in Qi activity. Clinical manifestations such as collapse or coma will present in severe cases.

Qi block is the pathological state showing extreme Qi stagnation. Turbid Qi is expelled outward, thus blocking the outflow of Qi, which is often manifested as sudden coma.

Qi collapse can be caused either by weakened antipathogenic Qi, which fails in guarding the interior, or profuse sweating or long-term loss of Blood which causes collapse of Qi and Blood. It is often seen in a sudden decline in the functions of the human body.

3. DEFICIENCY OF BLOOD

This refers to the pathological condition of malnutrition in the Zang Fu organs, meridians and collaterals which is due to insufficient Blood supply, thus failing to offer nourishment and moisture.

Formation: Hypofunction in Blood production, excessive Blood loss, consumption of Essence and Blood due to prolonged illness or over-exhaustion can all result in deficiency of Blood.

Clinical manifestations: When Blood is not sufficient to nourish the muscle and skin, there will be symptoms such as pallor or yellowish complexion, rough skin, dry hair, pale tongue and white coating.

Insufficient Blood supply to the head may also lead to dizziness and vertigo.

When Blood cannot nourish the eyes there will be blurred vision and night blindness.

If Blood fails to nourish tendons, numbness of hand and foot, motor impairment of the four limbs and spasm may present.

When Blood fails to nourish the nails, the nails will be pale and easily broken.

Insufficient Blood supply to the Heart may result in palpitations.

If Blood cannot nourish the Mind, mental activity will be disturbed. Symptoms such as mental derangement, irritability, dream-disturbed sleep, poor memory, difficulty in concentration and restlessness may occur.

4. STAGNATION OF THE BLOOD

Stagnation of the Blood refers to an accumulation of Blood due to hindrance to the Blood circulation.

Formation: Stagnation of Qi obstructs Blood circulation, or deficiency of Qi slows down Blood circulation. Furthermore, stagnation of Blood can also be caused by turbid Phlegm obstructing the meridians and collaterals. Other causative factors can be Cold attacking Blood or Heat attacking Blood. Blood stasis is the pathological product coming from unsmooth circulation of the Blood; however, Blood stasis may obstruct the Qi and Blood circulation, which conversely may lead to the formation of Blood stasis.

Clinical manifestations: If Blood obstructs at a local region, there will be pain with fixed location, formation of mass, and pain that cannot be relieved by Cold or warmth. Other symptoms are ecchymosis or petechia, purple lips, and dark tongue. It is therefore obvious that Blood stasis may disturb Qi activity, and Qi stagnation will influence Blood circulation.

5. HEAT IN THE BLOOD

Heat in the Blood refers to the pathological state of Blood disturbance, or accelerated Blood circulation.

Formation: Invasion of Heat to the Blood or transformation of endogenous pathogenic Heat into Fire, which attacks the Blood.

Clinical manifestations: Signs of Heat, consumption of Blood, bleeding, and consumption of Yin.

6. DYSFUNCTION OF QI AND BLOOD

As discussed earlier in this book, Qi is the commander of Blood, and Blood is the mother of Qi. The relationship between Qi and Blood can be concluded as being interpromoting, interdependent, and intertransforming. Qi mainly provides warmth and motiving force, whilst Blood provides nourishment and moisture. A dysfunction of Qi and Blood is mainly manifested as stagnation of Qi and Blood, with Qi failing to control Blood, collapse of Qi with Blood, deficiency of Qi and Blood, and Qi and Blood failing to nourish the meridians, etc.

6.1 Stagnation of Qi and Blood

Stagnation of Qi and Blood refers to the pathological state due to the irregular circulation of Qi and Blood. Since the Heart-Qi dominates Blood circulation, the Liver-Qi takes charge of the free flow of the Qi of the entire body, and the Liver stores Blood. Therefore stagnation of Qi and Blood are closely related to dysfunctions of the Liver and Heart. Clinical manifestations are mainly seen as distention and pain, ecchymosis, and mass in the abdomen.

6.2 Qi fails in controlling Blood

This refers to the pathological state when Qi is too weak to control Blood circulating normally inside the bood vessels, and so extravasation occurs.

6.3 Qi collapse with Blood

This refers to the pathological state showing as deficiency of Qi and Blood, or collapse of Qi and Blood. In cases of massive bleeding, there will also be loss of Qi, which is described as 'Qi follows Blood in becoming exhausted'.

6.4 Deficiency of Qi and Blood

This refers to the pathological state showing as the declined function of the human body; Qi deficiency and Blood deficiency existing at the same time. Clinical manifestations are mainly seen as pallor, or sallow complexion, lassitude, reluctance to speak, a thin body, palpitations, insomnia, dry skin and hair, and numbness of the four limbs.

6.5 Failure of Qi and Blood in nourishing the meridians

Failure of Qi and Blood in nourishing the meridians refers to the pathological state manifesting as malnutrition to bood vessels, tendons, muscles and skin, or motor impairment of limbs, which may be induced by the weakened function of Qi and Blood, or disharmony of Qi and Blood.

IV. DISORDERS OF BODY FLUID METABOLISM

Disorders in the formation, distribution and excretion of Body Fluids may lead to insufficient formation, and excessive loss of Body Fluid. Pathological changes such as overconsumption and retention of water within the body can be caused by inadequacy of Body Fluid or disturbance in distribution or excretion of Body Fluid.

The formation, distribution and excretion of Body Fluid depends on the ascending, descending, outward and inward movement of Qi, and the functional activities of Qi. Referring to the physiological functions of the Zang Fu organs, the formation of Body Fluid is closely related with the transformation and transportation functions of the Spleen and the Stomach. The distribution and excretion of Body Fluid cannot be completed without the function of the Spleen in dispersing the nutrient substances, the function of the Liver in maintaining the free flow of Qi, the function of the Triple Burner in regulating the water passage, the dispersing and descending function of the Lungs and the Qi activities of the Kidneys and the Bladder (see Figure 6.1).

Pathological changes that can occur include the following.

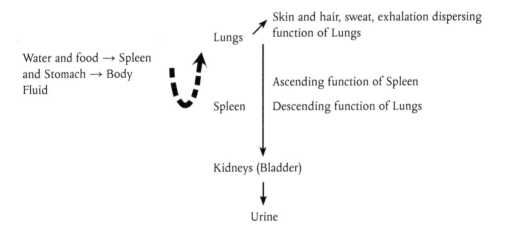

Figure 6.1: The distribution and excretion of Body Fluid

1. INSUFFICIENT BODY FLUID

An inadequacy of Body Fluid leads to a failure to moisten the Zang Fu organs, skin and hair, and all the tissues and organs throughout the body, and this leads to a series of pathological changes that are manifested by Dryness.

Aetiology and pathogenesis: Insufficient Body Fluid can result from the condensing of Body Fluid by exogenous pathogenic Heat and Dryness, or endogenous Heat due to emotional disorders. Overconsumption of Body Fluid can be caused by severe vomiting, diarrhoea, profuse sweating, frequent urination (with increased volume) and haemorrhage, etc. Improper intake of herbs that are pungent and dry in nature may also reduce the Body Fluid. Insufficient Body Fluid can also be seen in patients with chronic disease, whose body constitution is so weakened that it leads to disturbance in producing sufficient Body Fluid.

Clinical manifestations of overconsumption of 'Jin': Clear and thin Body Fluids are referred to as 'Jin' and overconsumption of this can lead to: profuse sweating in hot weather; thirst with a strong desire to drink due to high fever; dry mouth, nose and skin when exposed to the dry environment; sunken eyes and spasm caused by severe vomiting, diarrhoea and frequent urination (with increased volume), etc.

Clinical manifestations of overconsumption of 'Ye': Thick and heavy Body Fluids are known as 'Ye' and overconsumption of these can lead to manifestations such as: red and smooth tongue body without tongue-coating or with less coating, dry lips and tongue without the desire to drink, emaciation, haggard skin and hair, muscular twitching and cramp. Tremor of hands and feet can also be seen in the late phase of febrile diseases or in patients with chronic diseases.

2. DISTURBANCE IN THE DISTRIBUTION AND EXCRETION OF BODY FLUID

2.1 Disturbance in distribution of Body Fluid

This refers to disorders of transmission and distribution of Body Fluid. The retarded flow of Body Fluid or retention of Body Fluid at the local area may cause water and Damp retention in the interior, and finally lead to Phlegm retention.

Aetiology and pathogenesis: This is closely related to the dispersing and descending functions of the Lungs, the transportation and transformation functions of the Spleen, the function of the Liver in maintaining the free flow of Qi and the function of the Triple Burner in regulating the passage of water. Among these, a disorder of the transportation and transformation functions of the Spleen may have the most effect. *Plain Questions* states: 'Most of the problems caused by Damp retention, for instance, oedema, fullness and distention, are associated with the Spleen.' Disturbance in distribution of Body Fluid may lead to pathological changes such as Damp, Phlegm and water retention.

2.2 Disturbance in excretion of Body Fluid

Disturbance in excreting of Body Fluid refers to the pathological condition of water retention resulting from the failure of Body Fluid to transform into sweat or urine.

Aetiology and pathogenesis: Disturbance in excretion of Body Fluid is mainly related to the Lungs and the Kidneys. Qi activity of the Kidneys dominates excretion.

The transformation of Body Fluid into sweat mainly relies on the dispersing function of the Lungs, while the transformation of Body Fluid into urine depends on the Qi activity of the Kidneys. Dysfunction of the Lungs and the Kidneys can lead to Water retention with the major manifestation of oedema. The Qi activity of the Kidneys is the predominant factor for the excretion of Body Fluid. The book *Plain Questions* states: 'The Qi activity of the Kidneys in being in charge of excretion of urine and faeces makes the Kidneys act like the metabolic gate of the Stomach which takes in food and water. Dysfunction of the Kidneys may lead to water retention. When the retained water affects the skin, oedema will occur. Oedema is caused by retention of Body Fluid.'

Disturbance in distribution and excretion of Body Fluid interact as both cause and effect. They affect each other, and together can lead to pathological changes such as retention of Damp, Phlegm and water.

3. THE RELATIONSHIP BETWEEN QI, BLOOD AND BODY FLUID

The formation, distribution and excretion of Body Fluid depend upon the Qi activities of the Zang Fu organs as well as the ascending, descending, outward and inward movement of Qi. Body Fluid acts as the carrier of Qi, which can distribute Qi throughout the body. Sufficient Body Fluid can fill up the bood vessels and maintain the free flow of Blood. Pathological changes due to dysfunction of Body Fluid, Qi and Blood can be seen as the follows.

3.1 Qi stagnation due to Body Fluid retention

This refers to the pathological condition of Qi stagnation resulting from water, Dampness and Phlegm retention caused by disturbance of Body Fluid metabolism. For instance, dampness retention in the Lungs may lead to Lung-Qi stagnation. This impairs the dispersing and descending functions of the Lungs. The clinical manifestations of this can be seen as fullness in the chest, cough, and asthma which is worse on lying flat. An attack on the Heart by retained fluid may block Heart-Qi circulation and inhibit Heart Yang, the clinical manifestations of which can be palpitation and cardiac pain. Excessive fluid in the Middle Burner can cause dysfunction of the Spleen and the Stomach so that the clear Qi fails to ascend and the turbid Qi cannot descend. Clinical manifestations in this situation can be mental cloudiness, lassitude, fullness and distention in the epigastric region and poor appetite, while accumulation of water and Dampness at the four extremities which blocks the Qi and Blood circulation in meridians may result in heaviness and distending pain in the limbs.

3.2 Exhaustion of Qi resulting from excessive loss of Body Fluid

This refers to the pathological condition where excessive loss of Body Fluid leads to massive dissipation of Qi. This overconsumption of Body Fluid can be the result of high fever, profuse sweating, severe vomiting and diarrhoea.

3.3 Exhaustion of both Body Fluid and Blood

This refers to the pathological condition of generation of a deficiency type of Heat in the interior of the body or stirring up of interior Wind resulting from exhaustion of Body Fluid and Blood. Body Fluid and Blood are of the same origin. This syndrome often results from overconsumption of Body Fluid due to high fever or burn, excessive loss of Body Fluid by haemorrhage or hectic fever caused by Yin deficiency. It gives rise to the clinical manifestations of irritability, dry nose and throat, feverish sensations in the Five Centres, emaciation, scaley and dry skin, itching of the skin and desquamation, etc.

3.4 Blood stagnation due to insufficient Body Fluid

This refers to the pathological condition of blockage of Blood circulation resulting from overconsumption of Body Fluid. High fever, burns, vomiting, diarrhoea and profuse sweating are the main causes. Excessive loss of Body Fluid leads to decreased Blood volume and poor Blood circulation, which may finally result in Blood stagnation. This gives rise to those clinical manifestations of insufficient Body Fluid, and at the same time, may be accompanied by a purplish tongue with dark spots, or mucular eruption.

V. INTERIOR PATHOGENIC FACTORS

The five interior pathogenic factors: This refers to the pathological phenomenon resulting from disorders of Qi, Blood, and Body Fluid, and dysfunction of the

Zang Fu organs, which appear during the progress of diseases. The characteristics of diseases caused by the five interior pathogenic factors, namely 'interior Wind', 'interior Cold', 'interior Dampness', 'interior Dryness' and 'interior Fire', are similar to those caused by five of the six exogenous pathogenic factors, that is, Wind, Cold, Dampness, Dryness and Fire. The five interior pathogenic factors are not actually causative factors of diseases, but a kind of comprehensive pathological change resulting from disorders of Qi, Blood, Body Fluid and dysfunction of the Zang Fu organs.

1. STIRRING UP OF INTERIOR WIND

1.1 Concept

Stirring up of interior Wind, or 'interior Wind' in short, is mostly related to the Liver. It is often called 'stirring up of the Liver Wind interiorly'. During the progress of disease, symptoms such as vertigo and dizziness, convulsion and tremor may appear when there is a predominance of Yang, or a hyperactivity of Yang due to the failure of Yin to control Yang. These are all manifestations of stirring up of interior Wind, the pathological condition resulting from hyperactivity of Yang internally.

1.2 Pathogenesis

1.2.1 Wind syndrome due to hyperactivity of Liver Yang

This refers to the pathological condition resulting from Liver and Kidney Yin deficiency which give rise to hyperactivity of Liver Yang. It indicates the impairment of Water to nourish Wood according to the Theory of the Five Elements. In mild cases, symptoms of mental cloudiness, blurred vision, numbness of the extremities, carebaria, tremor of hands and feet, vertigo and dizziness may occur. In severe cases, there can be sudden loss of consciousness (which is the manifestation of the adverse flow of Qi and Blood), deviation of mouth and eyes, hemiplegia, and critical syndromes such as excess syndrome of apoplectic coma or prostration syndrome, etc.

1.2.2 Occurrence of Wind syndrome in cases of extreme Heat

This is a pathological condition of the occurrence of Wind syndrome resulting from the hyperactivity of Yang due to an attack of pathogenic Heat which scorches the Liver meridian. Its clinical manifestations can be: convulsions, contraction, flaring of nostrils, staring up of the eyes, opisthotonos, and accompanied by symptoms indicating disturbance of Mind by Heat, such as high fever, mental cloudiness and delirium.

1.2.3 Occurrence of Wind syndrome due to Yin deficiency

This refers to a pathological condition of the occurrence of Wind syndrome caused by Liver and Kidney Yin deficiency. The clinical manifestations can be tremor of the hands and feet, muscular twitching and cramp, accompanied by Yin deficiency manifestations such as dry mouth, emaciation, low fever, feverish sensation in the Five Centres, dry tongue, and a thready and rapid pulse.

1.2.4 Occurrence of Wind syndrome due to Blood deficiency

This refers to a pathological condition of the occurrence of a deficiency type of Wind syndrome resulting from Liver Blood deficiency, which cannot nourish the meridians and collaterals. The clinical manifestations can be numbness of the extremities, muscle spasm, and motor impairment of fingers and toes with muscular constriction, accompanied by manifestations of Blood deficiency such as a lustreless face, vertigo and dizziness, pale tongue and a thready pulse.

2. PRODUCTION OF INTERIOR COLD

2.1 Concept

Production of interior Cold is also called 'interior Cold' for short. It is a pathological condition involving generation of a deficiency type of Cold internally or a predominance of Yin, which results from the deficient Yang Qi failing to complete its warming-up function.

2.2 Pathogenesis

- Yang deficiency fails to warm up the body and results in predominance of Yin, which produces interior Cold. Contraction of bood vessels may slow down the Blood circulation. This gives rise to clinical manifestations such as pale complexion, Cold limbs, muscle spasm, and pain in the extremities, etc. Generation of interior Cold has the closest association with Spleen and Kidney Yang deficiency. The Spleen dominates the four extremities, and Spleen Yang can reach and warm up the muscles on the extremities. Kidney Yang is the foundation of the Yang Qi in the human body. It can warm up the Zang Fu organs and tissues throughout the body. So the manifestations of deficiency type of Cold may appear to be due to Yang Qi deficiency of the Spleen and the Kidneys, especially due to Kidney Yang deficiency which fails to warm up the body.

- Yang-Qi deficiency can impair the Qi activity and cause metabolism disturbance, which may ultimately cause retention of the pathological productions that are Yin and Cold in nature, such as Dampness and Phlegm. Yang Qi deficiency can give rise to the clinical manifestations of frequent urination with clear and increased volume, clear and thin nasal discharge and sputum, or diarrhoea and oedema.

2.3 Interior Cold and exterior Cold

From clinical manifestations, 'interior Cold' is a deficiency type of Cold with mainly deficiency manifestations, whilst 'exterior Cold' is characterized chiefly by Cold, or may be accompanied by some deficiency manifestations, but still takes Cold as its major property. The relationship between these two can be manifested as follows: invasion by an exogenous Cold pathogenic factor may lead to damage of Yang Qi and cause Yang deficiency, while a Yang-deficient body constitution with declined ability to resist pathogenic factors will easily be affected again by an exterior Cold pathogenic factor.

3. PRODUCTION OF INTERIOR DAMP

3.1 Concept

Production of interior Damp is also called 'interior Damp' for short. It is a pathological condition of Damp and Phlegm retention due to impairment of the transportation and transformation functions of the Spleen.

3.2 Pathogenesis

The causative factors of Damp retention due to Spleen deficiency can be an excessively Damp and Phlegmy body constitution, which is often seen in obese patients, and dysfunction of the Spleen and the Stomach due to over-eating raw, cold or greasy food. The Spleen loses its transportation and transformation functions, which cause a disturbance in distribution of Body Fluid, and finally leads to Damp and Phlegm retention. Kidney Yang is the foundation of all kinds of Yang in the human body and Kidney Yang deficiency impairs the transportation and transformation functions of the Spleen and gives rise to interior Damp. Conversely, Damp is a kind of Yin pathogenic factor that easily damages Yang Qi. Chronic Damp retention can cause Spleen and Kidney Yang Qi deficiency, which again results in excessive Damp accumulation. Damp is characterized by heaviness, turbidity and stickiness, which easily obstructs Qi circulation. Clinical manifestations vary according to the area of the body affected.

- **Retained Dampness attacking the superficial part of the body**: A heavy sensation in the head as though it has been wrapped in a piece of cloth, heaviness of the body as though it were carrying a heavy load.

- **Accumulation of Dampness in joints**: Sensation of heaviness in the joints, or motor impairment of joints.

- **Retention of Dampness in the Upper Burner**: Fullness in the chest, cough with profuse and sticky sputum.

- **Retention of Dampness in the Middle Burner**: Fullness in the epigastric region, poor appetite, sticky sensation or sweet taste in mouth, thick and sticky tongue-coating.

- **Retention of Dampness in the Lower Burner**: Fullness and distention in abdomen, loose stools, dysuria.

- **Accumulated Dampness affecting the skin**: Oedema.

3.3 Exterior Dampness and interior Dampness

Invasion by an exterior Dampness pathogenic factor may often damage the function of the Spleen. When the Spleen loses its transportation and transformation functions, there will be Dampness generated internally. In the clinic, a Dampness retention body constitution which is due to dysfunction of the Spleen in transportation and transformation can very easily be further attacked by exterior Dampness, which will cause exaggerated symptoms.

4. DRYNESS DUE TO OVERCONSUMPTION OF BODY FLUID

4.1 Concept

This refers to a pathological condition manifested by symptoms that are of Dryness in nature. It results from insufficient Body Fluid, which fails to nourish the organs and tissues throughout the body.

4.2 Pathogenesis

Overconsumption of the Body Fluid can be caused by chronic diseases that consume the Yin fluid and lead to profuse sweating, severe vomiting, and diarrhoea. Haemorrhage can lead to insufficient of Yin fluid in the body. Consumption of Body Fluid can result from excessive Heat due to febrile diseases. Pathogenic Dampness can also transform into Dryness. Insufficient Body Fluid fails to moisten the Zang

Fu organs, skin, and orifices of the body, and thus Dryness and Heat are generated. Clinical manifestations can be seen as: dry and lustreless skin, desquamation, cracks in the skin, dry throat and mouth, cracked lips, dry tongue or red cracked tongue without tongue-coating, dry nose and eyes, broken and brittle nails, constipation, scanty and yellowish urination, etc. Dryness in the Lungs results in cough without sputum, or with sputum that is difficult to spit out, or even haemoptysis. Dryness attacks the Stomach, which may cause Stomach Yin deficiency and leads to red tongue without coating, while Dryness of the intestines gives rise to constipation.

5. GENERATION OF INTERIOR FIRE

5.1 Concept

This is a pathological condition that refers to hyperfunction of the body due to internal Fire. Qi or Blood stagnation or chronic diseases can cause excessive Yang or hyperactivity of Yang due to Yin deficiency, and further generates Fire internally. 'Interior Fire' is often also described as 'internal Heat'.

5.2 Pathogenesis

5.2.1 Transformation of excessive Yang Qi into Fire

Yang Qi has the function of warming up the body, promoting the functions of the Zang Fu organs, and the tissues and activating Qi and Blood circulation. It is often known as 'physiological Fire'. Under pathological conditions, excessive Yang Qi may lead to hyperactivity of the Zang Fu organs and overconsumption of Yin fluid. In these circumstances, the excessive Yang Qi is called 'exaggerated pathologic Fire'. It says that 'excess Qi can be called Fire'.

5.2.2 Transformation of retained pathogenic factors into Fire

This is a pathological condition of transformation of Fire-Heat from interior retention of the six exogenous pathogenic factors, that is, Wind, Cold, Dryness and Dampness, etc. For instance, Cold retention can transform into Heat, while dampness retention can transform into Fire. Retention of the pathological products such as Phlegm, stagnated Blood, retained food or parasites can block Qi circulation and can also transform it into Fire.

5.2.3 Fire caused by emotional disorders

Emotional stress, mental stimulations, disorder of the Qi and Blood and dysfunction of the Zang Fu organs can result in Qi stagnation. Prolonged Qi stagnation may transform into Heat, thus generating Fire Heat. Clinically, emotional depression often leads to Liver-Qi stagnation which may transform into Fire. The manifestations of 'Liver Fire' can be irritability, redness of the eyes and hot temper, etc.

5.2.4 Hyperactivity of Fire due to Yin deficiency

A deficiency type of Heat or Fire can be produced due to hyperactivity of Yang that results from insufficient Yin fluid and overconsumption of Blood. Fever of deficiency type such as tidal fever, a feverish sensation in the Five Centres and night sweating can be seen in general. Heat or Fire manifestations such as toothache, sore throat, dry mouth and lips and flushed cheeks due to flaring-up of the deficiency type of Fire can be seen in localized areas.

VI. PATHOGENESIS ACCORDING TO THE MERIDIANS AND COLLATERALS

This refers to pathological changes due to the attack on the meridian system by pathogenic factors directly or indirectly. These pathological changes are mainly reflected in an excess or deficiency of Qi and Blood in the meridians and collaterals, a disorder of Qi and Blood circulation in the meridians and collaterals, Qi and Blood stagnation in the meridians and collaterals, and exhaustion of Qi and Blood in the meridians and collaterals, etc.

CHAPTER 7

PREVENTION OF DISEASES AND PRINCIPLES OF TREATMENT

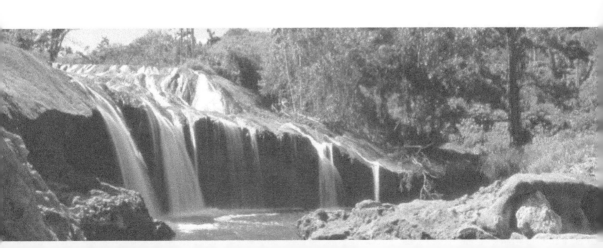

I. PREVENTION

1. CONCEPTS AND PRINCIPLES OF TREATMENT

Prevention refers to the adoption of certain measures to prevent the occurrence and progress of diseases.

Principles of treatment: Prevention before the attack of a disease, and prevention from deterioration after occurrence of a disease.

1.1 Prevention before the attack of a disease

Prevention before the attack of a disease refers to the adoption of various preventative methods before the occurrence of a disease, as described below.

1.1.1 Keeping healthy, and enhancing the ability of the body to resist pathogenic factors

Building up the body resistance is the key point in enhancing the ability of body resistance to resist pathogenic factors. Attention should be paid to emotional regulation, physical exercise, diet, lifestyle and avoidance of overstrain and stress. Appropriate drug prophylaxis can be applied as well.

Emotional regulation: Sudden and strong emotional stimulation or persistent and repeated mental stimulation can cause disease due to derangement of Qi circulation, and disorders of Qi, Blood and Yin–Yang. Emotional stimulation can lead to weakness of the antipathogenic Qi, which gives a chance for the invasion of exterior pathogenic factors. In the progress of diseases, emotional disturbance can further exacerbate the disease. So, regulating emotions may reinforce the ability of the antipathogenic Qi to resist diseases, thus preventing the occurrence of disease.

Strengthening physical training: Exercise makes for a vigorous life, and health relies on physical training. To strengthen physical training is to reinforce body constitution. This is a very important action in decreasing and preventing the occurrence of disease.

A regular lifestyle: Health care that follows the laws of nature can guarantee a vigorous and lengthened life. So, appropriate attention should be paid to diet, exercise and rest in order to regulate the lifestyle.

Drug prophylaxis and artificial immunization: Great importance has been attached to prevention using Chinese herbal medicine, and significant development has been made in this aspect.

1.1.2 Preventing the attack of pathogenic factors

Pathogenic factors are major factors that may cause disease. Besides reinforcing the body constitution and strengthening the antipathogenic Qi, importance should also be attached to preventing the attack of pathogenic factors. For instance, attention should be paid to hygiene. Environmental pollution, water and food contamination should be avoided. Traumatic injury, insect and animal bites should be avoided as well as far as possible.

1.2 Prevention from deterioration after the occurrence of a disease

Prevention from deterioration after the occurrence of a disease: Importance should be attached to early diagnosis and treatment of a disease in order to prevent its negative development.

1.2.1 Early diagnosis

If the invading exterior pathogenic factors cannot be eliminated in time, they may transform step by step from the superficial part of the body to the interior, and eventually affect the viscera. Disease may then become more complicated, severe and difficult to cure. The principles of occurrence and progress of diseases should be mastered in order to make early diagnoses, and give effective treatment and to prevent deterioration of the disease.

1.2.2 To reinforce the possibly affected area in advance according to the progressive law of diseases

For instance, *Classic on Medical Problems* states:

> If the Liver is diseased, attention should be paid to the Spleen, because Liver problems may affect the Spleen according to the Theory of the Five Elements. So the Spleen should be strengthened in advance to prevent the attack of the Spleen by the Liver.

According to this progress and prevention principle, prescriptions or medicines that have the function of consolidating the Spleen and regulating the function of the Stomach should be combined with the treatment of the Liver.

II. PRINCIPLES OF TREATMENT

Principles of treatment: The general principles of treatment are based on the concept of holistic treatments, and differentiation of syndromes. They are of universal significance in decisions concerning methods of treatment, prescriptions and medicines.

Therapeutic methods: Therapeutic methods are specific treatment methods directed toward manifestations and syndromes which are worked out within the guidance of the general principles. They have clear targets and can be applied flexibly. For instance, 'treating the same disease with different methods' and 'treating different diseases with the same therapeutic principle' embody the flexible application of the specific therapeutic methods.

Relationship between principles of treatment and therapeutic methods: Principles of Treatment refer to the general laws of treatment, whilst therapeutic methods are specific treatment methods which fall within the guidance of the general principles of treatment. In terms of pathogenic factors and the antipathogenic Qi, disease can reflect the predominance or weakness of pathogenic factors or antipathogenic Qi. Thus, here one must make the reinforcement of the antipathogenic Qi and the elimination of pathogenic factors the basic treating principle. Under the guidance of this principle, methods such as tonifying Qi, nourishing Blood and Yin, and reinforcing Yang should be adopted for different deficiency syndromes in order to reinforce the antipathogenic Qi. Therapeutic methods such as diaphoresis, Heat clearing, Blood activation, emetics and purgation can be adopted for various excess syndromes in order to eliminate pathogenic factors.

1. SETTING UP THE PRINCIPLES OF TREATMENT

Setting up the principles of treatment takes differentiation of syndromes as the essential prerequisite. The general law of treatment should be established on the basis of causative factors, location, property of the disease and conflict between pathogenic factors and antipathogenic Qi – which are summarized from the information collected by the four diagnostic methods.

2. APPLICATION OF THE PRINCIPLES OF TREATMENT

Treatment laws should be applied with flexibility and according to the established principles. For a simple syndrome, a single principle can be adopted, while towards a complicated syndrome, two or more principles should be combined and applied together. In different phases of the progress of the disease, various principles should be adopted to adapt to different natures.

2.1 Searching for the primary cause of disease in treatment

This is the basic law for diagnosis and treatment based on overall analysis of symptoms and signs. Occurrence and progress of disease is the process of conflict between pathogenic factors and antipathogenic Qi. Contradictions in the body are usually not alone. Clinical manifestations can reflect the principle contradiction in the body but sometimes may not do so. Proper treatment can only be given when a clear distinction can be drawn between the manifestations of the disease and the root cause of the disease, and when the principle aspect of the contradiction and the secondary aspect of the contradiction are distinguished. The instructions 'Routine treatment', 'treating a disease contrary to the routine' and the treating principle of 'treating the symptoms first when they are acute, and treating the root cause when these symptoms are relieved' embody the basic law of searching for the primary cause of disease in treatment.

2.1.1 Routine treatment and treating a disease contrary to the routine

Plain Questions states:

> Routine treatment is given according to the accepted view that treating methods are applied that have properties opposite to those of the symptoms. While treating a disease contrary to the routine seems to be adopted in opposition to the accepted view, here treating methods having similar characteristics with the property of the false manifestations are used.

Both approaches give expression to the principle of searching for the primary cause of disease in treatment.

Routine treatment: Through analysis of the clinical manifestations, the nature of the disease, such as Cold, Heat, deficiency or excess, should be distinguished, and various therapeutic methods be adopted – such as 'treating the Cold-syndrome with Hot-natured drugs', 'treating the Heat-syndrome with Cold-natured drugs', 'illness of deficiency type should be treated by tonifying method' and 'excess syndromes should be treated with the method of purgation and reduction', etc. Because the treatment is given according to the routine thought pattern, it is often know as 'routine treatment'.

Treating a disease contrary to the routine: This is a treating method that has the same characteristics as the properties of the false manifestations of the disease. Because the treatment that is given seems to be opposite to the routine thought pattern, it is often known as 'treating a disease contrary to the routine'. The following four points all pertain to the principle of treating a disease contrary to the routine:

- *Using medicine of a warm nature to treat pseudo-Heat syndrome*: This means using medicine of a warm nature to treat diseases Cold in nature but with Heat manifestations. It can be applied to Cold syndrome with pseudo-Heat symptoms resulting from predominance of Cold or Yin in the interior.

- *Using medicine of a Cold nature to treat pseudo-Cold syndrome*: Using medicine of a Cold nature to treat disease this is hot in nature but with Cold manifestations. It can be applied to Heat syndrome with pseudo-Cold symptoms resulting from predominance of Heat or Yang in the interior.

- *Treating obstructive diseases by tonification*: Using the reinforcing method to remove obstruction means using medicine with a tonification function to treat diseases of deficiency with symptoms of obstruction. They can be applied to what is a syndrome of deficiency in reality but that has pseudo-excess symptoms such as obstruction caused by a weak body constitution or hypofunction of the Zang Fu organs, Qi and Blood.

- *Treating diarrhoea with purgatives*: This refers to adopting purgatives instead of astringents to treat excess syndrome with symptoms of diarrhoea.

2.1.2 Treating symptoms and treating the root cause of disease

Although 'searching for the primary cause of disease in treatment' is the law in clinical treatment, under certain circumstances, the symptoms are very critical: if they cannot be treated immediately, they will affect the treatment of the root cause or perhaps even cause death. In such cases, it is necessary to observe the principle of 'treating the symptoms first when they are acute, and treating the root cause when these symptoms are relieved.' But if the primary and secondary aspects are both serious, they must be treated at the same time.

Treating the symptoms first when they are acute: Generally speaking, the principle contradiction leading to treating contrary to the routine and the main focus of a contradiction should be the root cause of the disease, not the symptoms. So searching for and treating the primary cause is the basic law in treatment. But, as mentioned above, under certain conditions, the symptoms are very critical and if not treated immediately, they will affect the treatment of the root cause or perhaps cause death. In this case, it is necessary to observe the principle of 'treating the symptoms first when they are acute, and treating the root cause when these symptoms are relieved'. For instance, with patients who are haemorrhaging, no matter what the causative reason, proper measures should be adopted immediately to stop the bleeding, which is taken as the symptom. When the bleeding has stopped, treatment should be given to relieve the root cause. Another example, with patients with chronic disease attacked by exterior pathogenic factors, if the symptoms caused by exterior pathogenic factors are acute, priority should be given to eliminating the exterior pathogenic factors to relieve the acute symptoms. Then, treatment can be focused on chronic diseases so as to treat the root cause. Treatment for the symptoms cannot be given persistently lest the antipathogenic Qi is damaged.

Treating the root cause when the acute symptoms are relieved: Under normal circumstances, treatment should be focused on the nature of the disease and measures should be adopted toward the root cause in particular. For instance, tuberculosis of the Lungs can be caused by interior Heat resulting from Yin deficiency. Cough, low fever, dry mouth and throat, a feverish sensation in the Five Centres, flushed cheeks and night sweating are its clinical manifestations, while interior Heat in Lungs due to Yin deficiency is the root cause. Thus, principles of treatment such as nourishing Yin and moistening the Lungs should be adopted so that here the treatment could be focused on the nature or the root cause of this disease.

Treating the root cause and the symptoms at the same time: When symptoms are very strong, and the syndrome is also critical, the principle of treating the root cause and the symptoms at the same time should be adopted. Take febrile disease caused by exterior pathogenic Heat, for example. Invasion of the exterior Heat pathogenic factor together with the interior excessive Heat which cannot be relieved in time may overconsume the Yin fluid. Clinical manifestations can be abdominal pain and distention, constipation, fever, dry mouth with cracked lips and a dry tongue-coating. For this syndrome with acute symptoms due to weakness of antipathogenic Qi and predominance of pathogenic factors, the principle of treating its symptoms and cause at the same time should be adopted. Purgation and nourishment of Yin could be applied at the same time so as to treat the root cause by clearing the Heat and relieving the acute symptoms by nourishing Yin. If only purgation is adopted, the Yin fluid may be further consumed, while if nourishing Yin is adopted on its own, it is not enough to clear the excessive Heat in the interior. The two may supplement each other in this case. Clearing Heat can help to reserve Yin, whilst nourishing Yin may assist to moisten the Dryness and promote defecation.

2.2 Strengthening body resistance and eliminating pathogenic factors

2.2.1 Strengthening the body resistance

This refers to reinforcing the antipathogenic Qi, building up health, and enhancing the ability of the body to resist pathogenic factors and to work towards rehabilitation. The principle can be applied to various deficiency diseases: 'Illness of deficiency type should be treated by tonifying method.' Therapeutic methods such as invigorating Qi, nourishing the Blood, nourishing Yin, warming Yang, replenishing Essence and tonifying the Zang Fu organs are all set up according to the principle of strengthening body resistance. Besides herbal decoctions, other treatments include acupuncture and moxibustion, Tuina, Qigong, diet therapy, emotional regulation and physical exercises, etc.

2.2.2 Eliminating the pathogenic factors

This includes eliminating the pathogenic factors, stopping the invasion of pathogenic factors and their damage to the body, and decreasing the hyperactive pathological responses of the body. The principle can be applied in various excess syndromes: 'Excess syndromes should be treated with the method of purgation and reduction.' Therapeutic methods such as diaphoresis, emetic therapy, purgation, removing food retention and promoting digestion, resolving Phlegm, promoting Blood circulation, dispelling Cold, clearing Heat and eliminating dampness are all set up according to the principle of eliminating the pathogenic factors.

Reinforcing the antipathogenic Qi can strengthen the body resistance, and may help in the elimination of pathogenic factors. It is said that 'once the body resistance against disease is strengthened, the pathogenic factors are removed.' To eliminate the pathogenic factors can decrease their damage to the body resistance, and this is expressed as 'once the pathogenic factors are removed, the body resistance will be reinforced.' Since they are closely related to each other, strengthening the body resistance is beneficial to dispelling the pathogenic factors, and vice versa.

2.2.3 Strengthening body resistance aiming at preventing the attack of pathogenic factors or eliminating the invaded pathogenic factors

Aiming at eliminating pathogenic factors and recuperating, treating therapies such as medicine, alimentotherapy, and dirigation should be adopted to strengthen body's resistance and enhance the restorative ability of the body. This is expressed as the concepts 'strengthening body resistance to eliminate pathogenic factors' and 'once the pathogenic factors are removed, the body resistance will be reinforced.'

The main step to strengthening body resistance is to tonify the deficient. The principle of reinforcing the deficient can be applied when the antipathogenic Qi is weak, while the pathogenic factors are not strong enough to overcome it, or when the principle contradiction, or the main aspect of the contradiction, lies in the weak antipathogenic Qi, while the attack of exterior pathogenic factors is just the secondary reason.

2.2.4 Eliminating the pathogenic factors aiming at strengthening the body resistance

Aiming at making the body restore its resistance to exterior pathogenic factors, treating therapies such as medicine, acupuncture and moxibustion, cupping or surgery could be applied to eliminate the pathogenic factors. This is expressed in the concepts 'eliminating pathogenic factors to assist strengthening body resistance' and 'once the pathogenic factors are removed, the body resistance will be reinforced.' This treating principle can be used for the condition when both pathogenic factor and antipathogenic Qi are strong, or when the principle contradiction, or the main aspect of the contradiction, focuses on the invasion of strong pathogenic factors with weakness of the antipathogenic Qi just as the secondary cause.

2.2.5 Attacking the pathogenic factors before tonifying

This is applicable in cases where driving out strong pathogenic factors is the first requirement and the pathogenic Qi is still strong enough to tolerate the eliminating method. Attacking the pathogenic factors before tonifying can be especially applied to weakness of antipathogenic Qi that directly results from an attack of pathogenic factors. For instance, in the case of febrile disease caused by exterior pathogenic factors, patients may have abdominal distention and pain, constipation due to Heat retention in the Stomach and intestines, red tongue, and black tongue-coating without moisture, dry mouth and throat, and even loss of consciousness with delirium, which result from overconsumption of Yin due to Heat retention in the interior. For such cases, attacking the pathogenic factors before tonifying should be used, and purgative therapy is applicable. Constipation may exaggerate the interior Heat retention, and further consume the Yin fluid, so purgation should be applied immediately to restore Yin, and medicine with the function of nourishing Yin and moistening the Dryness may be used afterwards.

2.2.6 Tonifying before attacking the pathogenic factors

This can be applied in cases where pathogenic factors are strong and at the same time antipathogenic Qi is so weak that Yin or Yang is exhausted. Because of the extreme weakness of antipathogenic Qi which cannot tolerate the drastic purgative method, tonifying before attacking the pathogenic factors should be adopted. When the antipathogenic Qi is consolidated, pathogenic factors can then be eliminated.

2.2.7 Reinforcing and eliminating in combination

This is a therapeutic method of strengthening the body resistance and eliminating the pathogenic factors at the same time. It is suitable in syndromes where there is weak antipathogenic Qi and an invasion of strong pathogenic factors. The predominant cause should be distinguished between antipathogenic Qi and pathogenic factors. If the attack of a strong pathogenic factor is the main reason, attention should be paid to eliminating pathogenic factors which will help to strengthen the antipathogenic Qi. Where there is extreme weakness of the antipathogenic Qi due to chronic diseases and at the same time incomplete elimination of pathogenic factors, priority should be given to strengthening body resistance, and proper consideration should also be given to driving out the pathogenic factors.

2.3 Regulating Yin-Yang

The occurrence of any diseases is, fundamentally speaking, due to the relative imbalance of Yin–Yang. The normal interconsuming-supporting relationship between Yin and Yang is disturbed by either preponderance or discomfiture of Yin or Yang. Regulation of Yin–Yang is therefore a fundamental principle in clinical treatment.

2.3.1 Removing the excess

The method of 'removing excess' or 'reducing the preponderance' can be used when regulating the predominance of Yin or Yang. Yang in excess makes Yin suffer and Yin in excess makes Yang suffer. Excessive Yang Heat is likely to injure Yin fluid, whilst excessive Yin Cold is likely to damage Yang Qi. On regulating the preponderance of Yin or Yang, attention should be paid to the condition as to whether a corresponding Yin or Yang deficiency exists. If one is deficient, consideration should be given to both Yin reduction and Yang reinforcement (or vice versa) simultaneously.

2.3.2 Reinforcing the deficient

The method of 'reinforcing the deficient' can be applied when regulating the deficiency of Yin or Yang. If both Yin and Yang are deficient, the reinforcing method should be adopted for both Yin and Yang. Attention should be paid to the principle of 'achieving Yin from Yang' or 'achieving Yang from Yin'. When strengthening Yin, medicine that has the function of tonifying Yang should be combined with it, and when tonifying Yang, medicine with the function of reinforcing Yin can be combined with it.

2.4 Regulation of the function of the Zang Fu organs

The human body is an organic entity. Physiologically, there is an interpromoting and coordination relationship between Zang and Zang organs, Zang and Fu organs, and also between Fu and Fu organs. Pathologically, dysfunction of the Zang Fu organs can affect each other. When a certain Zang or Fu organ is diseased, it may affect other Zang Fu organs. So, isolated treatment should not be given to a single Zang or Fu organ, but overall consideration should be given to regulating the comprehensive functions of the Zang Fu organs.

2.5 Regulating Qi and Blood

Qi and Blood are the material foundation of the functional activities of the body. Although Qi and Blood differ in their functions, they can promote each other and supplement the functions of each other. When there is a disorder of the interpromoting and interdepending relationship between Qi and Blood, syndromes due to derangement between Qi and Blood may occur. For instance:

- *Qi produces Blood.* Qi deficiency fails to produce sufficient Blood and results in Blood deficiency, and finally may cause deficiency of both Qi and Blood. Treatment should be focused on tonification of Qi, by assisting in the tonification and nourishment of Blood, not simply nourishing the Blood.

- *Qi can promote Blood circulation.* Qi deficiency or Qi stagnation may result in poor Blood circulation and Blood stagnation may follow. Principles of treatment such as promoting Blood circulation by reinforcing Qi or activating Blood circulation and removing stagnation by regulating Qi circulation can be adopted in this case.

- *Disorders of Qi can cause disorders of Blood circulation.* For instance, upward invasion of the hyperactive Liver-Qi often combines with upflow of Blood, and may result in loss of consciousness and haemoptysis. Sending down abnormal ascending Qi and adjusting the flow of Blood can be the proper treating principle in this situation.

- *Qi can control the Blood running inside the bood vessels.* Deficiency of Qi may impair its controlling function on Blood, leading to various types of haemorrhage. To stop a haemorrhage due to Qi deficiency, the method of tonifying Qi must be used.

- *Blood is the mother of Qi.* Blood deficiency may directly lead to Qi deficiency. Haemorrhage can result in exhaustion of Qi. According to the relation between Qi and Blood, tonification of Qi can be applied here to stop haemorrhages.

2.6 Treatment of diseases according to climatic and seasonal conditions, geographical locations and the individual conditions

The climatic and seasonal conditions, geographical location, patient's age and constitution must all be taken into consideration with determining an appropriate treating method. Among factors such as climatic and seasonal conditions, geographical location and individual constitutions, the last may have the strongest relation with the disease.

2.6.1 Treatment according to climatic and seasonal conditions

In accordance with the characteristics of climate and seasons, appropriate therapeutic methods are used. Generally, in spring and summer, the climate changes from warm to hot. Yang Qi is the predominant Qi. The skin and skin pores are open. Medicines that are pungent in flavour and warm in property should not be applied too extensively in any syndrome caused by exterior Wind Cold, so as to avoid the over-dispersing that may overconsume Qi and Yin. In autumn and winter, the climate changes from cool to cold. This leads to the predominance of Yin but the declining of Yang. Yang Qi is stored in the interior through the closing of skin and skin pores. Medicines that are bitter in taste and Cold in nature should be used very carefully to avoid damage of Yang. Diseases caused by Summer Heat are mainly seen in summertime, which is often characterized by high humidity. So, clearing away Summer Heat and eliminating Dampness can be the appropriate principles here. Dryness is predominant in autumn, so Dryness should be moistened with drugs that are pungent in flavor and cool in nature.

2.6.2 Treatment according to geographical location

The appropriate therapeutic methods should be determined according to the different geographical locations. Climate and lifestyle vary in different regions, as do physiological activities and pathological changes. Therefore, the methods of treatment and selection of medicine should be different.

2.6.3 Treatment according to individual conditions

The appropriate therapeutic methods should also be determined based on comprehensive consideration of age, gender, body constitution and lifestyle.

Age: Physiological conditions and the condition of Qi and Blood of people at different ages are different. Treatment and medicine should be given with consideration to age. Children are full of vigour and vitality, but their Zang Fu organs are delicate, Qi and Blood are not abundant, and their disease may be characterized by rapid changes and with manifestations of alternation of Cold and Heat, deficiency and excess. The dosage of drugs for infantile diseases should be small, and drastic purgation often be avoided. Young adults or middle-aged strong people are full of Qi and Blood, and the functions of their Zang Fu organs are active. Most of their diseases are an excess type due to violent conflict between the body resistance and pathogenic factors. Treatment can be focused on eliminating pathogenic factors and reducing excess, and the dosage can be increased. Vitality gradually decreases in older people, and their Qi and Blood decline as well. The properties of their diseases are mainly deficient or complicated deficiency and excess type. Principles of treatment such as reinforcing, or reinforcing and elimination in combination, are often followed.

Gender: Male and female are different in physiology. Females take Blood as their physiological foundation, and Liver as their most important organ, which can maintain the physiological activity of Blood. Pathologically, women can easily get problems associated with menstruation, leucorrhoea, pregnancy and puerperal conditions, as well as diseases related with the breasts and uterus. Drastic drugs with the functions of purgation, removing Blood stasis, promoting Blood circulation, inducing resuscitation and lubrication or toxic drugs should be used very carefully or are even contraindicated during the menstrual period and pregnancy. Elimination of Dampness can be applied for abnormal leucorrhoea, while for postpartum diseases, Qi and Blood deficiency or lochiorrhoea should be considered appropriate treatment. Males take Qi as their physiological foundation, and Kidneys as their congenital foundation. Pathologically, their Essence and Qi easily become deficient and this can cause sexual disorder. Treatment of problems such as impotence, priapism, prospermia, nocturnal emission, spermatorrhoea and gonic abnormality should be given based on the consideration of the Kidneys and other specific causes.

Body constitution: Basically, drugs or prescription that are warm or hot in nature should be avoided in patients with Yang-excess or Yin-deficiency body constitutions. Drugs or prescriptions that are Cool or Cold in nature should be avoided on patients with Yang-deficiency or Yin-excess body constitutions. Different patients with the same syndrome may be treated with different drugs. Attention should also be paid to career, working conditions, emotional factors and lifestyle during diagnosis and treatment.

GLOSSARY

Acronium A process on the shoulder blade.

Alimentotherapy Treatment of a condition by altering the diet.

Analgesia Reduced sensitivity to pain.

Anhidrosis The absence of perspiration where it should have been triggered.

Arthralgia Severe joint pain without swelling.

Ascariasis A genus of parasitic nematode worms.

Ascites Accumulation of fluid in the peritoneal cavity, resulting in abdominal swelling.

Auricular Of or relating to the ear or the sense of hearing.

Axilla The armpit.

Borborygmus Abdominal gurgling due to the movement of fluid and gas in the intestines.

Canthus Corner of the eye.

Cardia The opening between the oesophagus and the Stomach.

Carebaria Heavy headedness.

Cellulitis Inflammation of the skin caused by bacteria, often found on the lower legs.

Constringency Contracting or constraining.

Contracture The drawing together of skeletal muscle.

Costal Relating to the ribs.

Cubital fossa The depression at the front of the elbow.

Cun A Chinese unit of length. Traditionally equal to the width of a person's thumb at the knuckle, it has now been standardized to 3.33cm.

Cunkou Point on the radial artery at the wrist for pulse palpation.

Cyanosis A blue discoloration of the skin and mucous membranes caused by insufficient oxygen in blood vessels near the skin's surface.

Desquamation The removal of the outer layers of the skin by scaling.

Diaphoresis   Sweating or a treatment that causes sweating.

Dirigation   Development of control over functions that are usually involuntary.

Dorsum   The back. Also, the upper or posterior surface of a part of the body.

Dyspnoea   Difficulty breathing.

Dysuria   Difficult or painful urination.

Ecchymosis   A bruise.

Epicondyle   The protuberance above the protuberant end of an articulating bone.

Epigastrium   The central upper region of the abdomen.

Epiglottis   Thin flap of cartilage that lies behind the root of the tongue and covers the entrance to the larynx during swallowing.

Epistaxis   Bleeding from the nose.

Exogenous   Originating from outside the body.

Extensor pollicis brevis   A muscle in the thumb, which helps it to extend.

Extensor pollicis longus   A muscle in the thumb, which extends the thumb and works with the extensor pollicis brevis to extend the wrist.

Femoral artery   A large artery in the muscles of the thigh.

Frenulum   Folds of mucous membrane between the upper or lower lips and the gums, or under the tongue.

Flexor carpi radialis   A muscle in the forearm that acts to flex and abduct the hand.

Furuncle   A tender, pus-filled red lump caused by a skin infection. Also known as a boil.

Gastroptosis   The lowering, sinking or prolapse of the stomach.

Gluteal   Pertaining to the muscles of the buttocks.

Haematemesis   The vomiting of blood.

Haematochezia   The passing of bright red, bloody stools.

Haematuria   The passing of blood in the urine.

Haemoptysis   The coughing up of blood from the trachea, larynx, bronchi or lungs.

Hemiplegia   A condition involving the marked weakening of the limbs on one side of the body.

Humerus   The bone of the upper arm.

Hypochondrium   The upper lateral part of the abdomen, just beneath the lower ribs.

Ileocaecal conjunction   The valve between the small intestine and large intestine that prevents food from moving backwards into the small intestine.

Infraorbital region   The area below the eye.

Inguinal   Pertaining to the groin region.

Leucorrhoea   A discharge of mucus from the vagina.

Lochiorrhoea   The excessive discharge of blood, mucous and cell material through the vagina for an unusually long period of time after labour.

Mandible   The lower jawbone.

Medial malleolus   The inner ankle bone, at the lower end of the tibia.

Mentolabial groove   The groove on the chin below the lower lip.

Metacarpals   Bones of the hand.

Miasma   Harmful exhalations from rotting organic matter that pollute the atmosphere.

Nasopharynx   The part of the pharynx that connects to the nasal cavity.

Navicular bone   A bone of the ankle.

Occiput   The back of the head.

Oesophagus   The gullet – a tube that moves food from the mouth to the stomach.

Olecranon   The top part of the ulna, projects behind the elbow joint.

Opisthotonos   The position in which the head, neck and spine are arched backwards. In certain conditions this is involuntary.

Oxyuriasis   A common disease caused by the presence of a threadworm in the Large Intestine.

Palmaris longus   A muscle in the forearm that helps to flex the hand.

Parotitis   Inflammation of the salivary glands.

Perineum   Area of skin and muscle between the anus and the genitalia.

Petechiae   Small, round, flat, dark red spots caused by bleeding into the skin or underneath the mucous membranes.

Philtrum   The vertical groove on the median line of the upper lip.

Pisiform bone   The smallest bone of the wrist.

Polyhidrosis   Excessive and profuse perspiration.

Polylogia   Continuous and often incoherent speech.

Popliteus   A muscle at the back of the knee joint.

Priapism   Persistent and often painful penile erection requiring urgent medical treatment.

Prospermia   Premature ejaculation.

Pylorus   The lower end of the stomach. Ends in a ring of muscle that relaxes and contracts to control the passage of food and water to the Small Intestine.

Radius   The outer and shorter bone of the forearm.

Renalptosis   The lowering, sinking or prolapse of the kidney.

Scapula   Shoulder blade.

Spermatorrhoea   Excessive and involuntary discharge of semen without orgasm.

Stranguria   Severe pain in the urethra coming from the base of the bladder and associated with an intense desire to pass urine.

Styloid process   A spiny projection, e.g. at the lower end of the ulna.

Supraclavicular fossa   Indentation immediately above the collar bone.

Syncope   The loss of consciousness occurring when a sudden drop in blood pressure prevents sufficient blood flow to the brain. Also known as fainting.

Tenesmus   A frequent desire to defecate but without the production of significant amounts of faeces.

Thenar eminence   Group of muscles at the base of the thumb.

Tibia   Shin bone — the inner and larger bone of the lower leg.

Tidal fever   A fever that appears at the same time each day, and then declines.

Trismus   A spasm in the jaw muscles preventing the mouth from opening.

Tuberosity   Large, rounded protuberance on a bone.

Ulna   The inner and longer bone of the forearm.

Urticaria   An itchy rash with dark red raised bumps of which the cause may be allergic or non-allergic. Also known as hives.

Venule   A minute blood vessel.

Vertex   Centre of the top of the head — Baihui.

A BRIEF CHRONOLOGY OF THE CHINESE DYNASTIES

Dynasty		Time period
Xia		About 2100–1600 BCE
Shang		About 1600–1066 BCE
Zhou	Western Zhou	About 1066–771 BCE
	Eastern Xhou Spring and Autumn Period Warring States	About 770–256 BCE About 770–476 BCE About 475–221 BCE
Qin		About 221–206 BCE
Han	Western Han	About 206 BCE–23 CE
	Eastern Han	25–220 CE
Three Kingdoms	Wei	220–265 CE
	Shu	221–263 CE
	Wu	222–280 CE
Western Jin		265–316 CE
Eastern Jin Sixteen Kingdoms	Eastern Jin	317–420 CE
	Sixteen Kingdoms	304–439 CE

Northern and Southern	Southern	Song	420–479 CE
		Qi	479–502 CE
		Liang	502–557 CE
		Chen	557–589 CE
	Northern	Northern Wei	386–534 CE
		Eastern Wei	534–550 CE
		Northern Qi	550–577 CE
		Western Wei	535–557 CE
		Northern Zhou	557–581 CE
Sui			581–618 CE
Tang			618–907 CE
Five Dynasties and Ten Kingdoms	Later Liang		907–923 CE
	Later Tang		923–936 CE
	Later Jin		936–946 CE
	Later Han		947–950 CE
	Later Zhou		951–960 CE
	Ten Kingdoms		902–979 CE
Song	Northern Song		960–1127 CE
	Southern Song		1127–1279 CE
Liao			907–1125 CE
Western Xia			1038–1227 CE
Jin			1115–1234 CE
Yuan			1279–1368 CE
Ming			1368–1644 CE
Qing			1644–1911 CE
Republic of China			1912–1949 CE 1949–CE
People's Republic of China			1949 CE – present day

BIBLIOGRAPHY

Huang Di Nei Jing Su Wen (1979) 'Plain Questions.' *The Yellow Emperor's Classic of Internal Medicine.* Beijing: People's Health Publishing House.

Huang Di Nei Jing Ling Shu (1979) 'Miraculous Pivot.' *The Yellow Emperor's Classic of Internal Medicine.* Beijing: People's Health Publishing House.

Huang-fu Mi (1979) *Systematic Classic of Acupuncture and Moxibustion.* Bejing: People's Press.

Zhang Zhong Jing (2007) *Treatise on Febrile Diseases.* Translated by Luo Xiwen. Canada: Redwing Book Company.

INDEX